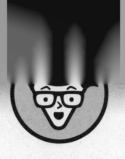

Intermittent Fasting

by Janet Bond Brill, PhD, RDN, FAND

Nationally recognized nutrition and fitness expert

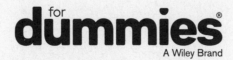

for **dummies**®

A Wiley Brand

Contents at a Glance

Recipes at a Glance

Table of Contents

PART 4: CUSTOMIZING YOUR COMPLETE INTERMITTENT FASTING PLAN

Introduction

Congratulations, you've come to the right place if you want to lose weight and body fat, get more fit, and improve your health! Fasting has been used throughout history to promote weight loss and increase longevity. Intermittent fasting, currently one of the world's most popular health and fitness trends, is a newer style of fasting that has gained considerable recognition in recent years, because many people find these regimens easier to follow than traditional, highly restrictive, calorie-counting diets. It's an uncomplicated concept, which makes it simple to follow without the deprivation associated with other diets. Translation: Intermittent fasting equals freedom! Intermittent fasting is not a diet in the conventional sense, but rather an eating pattern — a timed approach to eating.

That's why intermittent fasting has generated such a positive buzz — anecdotes of its effectiveness have proliferated around the globe. With intermittent fasting having become the go-to lifestyle, as a lifestyle research doctor, I needed to understand the science. So, I read the data and discovered a mountain of rock-solid scientific evidence showing that intermittent fasting, when combined with a healthy diet and lifestyle, is a remarkably effective approach for losing body fat, especially stubborn belly fat; maintaining or even gaining muscle; and treating or preventing many diseases and conditions that plague Americans.

What makes this health trend so popular? It's not really a diet, per se, but a new style of eating and living that after you get the hang of, it can allow you to attain your health and wellness goals and still embrace life and eat the delicious, healthy foods you love. You'll find out that it's not so much about what foods you should eat but more so, when you eat. As they say, "timing is everything."

About This Book

Intermittent Fasting For Dummies gives you all the tools you need to follow an intermittent fasting plan. Discover why simply changing the timing of your meals to allow for periodic breaks in eating can make such a positive difference in your body. With all the conflicting information about intermittent fasting out there, you may be wondering what's real and what's fake advice.

This handy guide puts all the important information together in plain English, laying out easy-to-follow guidelines for the different methods as well as describing what intermittent fasting can do for you — help you lose the fat for good, get healthier, fight disease, and hopefully increase your longevity. Remember, *you* are in charge, and you decide what will work for you.

By helping you eat fewer meals, intermittent fasting can lead to an automatic reduction in calorie intake. Additionally, it will positively change your hormone levels and flip the switch on your metabolism to facilitate all kinds of healthy bodily processes.

Specifically this book discusses the five most popular methods of intermittent fasting. Each type is effective, but may not be the right fit for everyone. You'll find out how to practice the different varieties of intermittent fasting as well as determine which method works best for your specific lifestyle.

This book is different from other books available about intermittent fasting because it's researched and written by a trusted expert in nutrition, health, and fitness — a registered dietitian and nutritionist — me! You can have confidence that the plans in this book are safe and based on sound science.

Foolish Assumptions

When writing this book, I made the following assumptions about you:

>> You may want to lose weight and keep it off.

>> You may want to get rid of excess body fat (especially stubborn belly fat).

>> You may already be lean and fit but want to tap into the myriad health benefits associated with intermittent fasting.

>> You want to increase your energy level and boost your metabolism.

>> You may have tried multiple diets in the past and been frustrated with the process and possibly gained back the weight.

>> You want to reduce the risk of diabetes, cancer, and heart disease.

>> You may want to simplify your life by freeing up time previously used to plan, cook, and clean up after all those meals.

>> You may have sensed all the excitement about intermittent fasting and want to give it a whirl.

>> You want to live a long, happy and healthy life.

Icons Used in This Book

Throughout this book, and in true *For Dummies* fashion, you'll notice several icons — all of them are designed to help you better understand and get the most out of your intermittent fasting plan. The following is a list of the icons you can expect to see throughout this book and what they mean:

TIP

This icon points to a tip that you can help your intermittent fasting process easier to follow.

REMEMBER

This piece of information is especially noteworthy and important.

WARNING

Warnings, if posted, are enormously significant. Be wary!

TECHNICAL STUFF

This book is based on scientific data and hypotheses, which may get a bit technical in the explanation. I hope to explain the scientific jargon in easy-to-grasp concepts, but if it's too confusing, skip it.

WEB EXTRAS

I'll occasionally direct you to a helpful website with this icon.

Beyond the Book

In addition to all the information in this book, you can find additional information online to help you with your intermittent fast. If you want to discover more about nutrition, healthy eating, and the Mediterranean Diet, you can visit my websites:

>> www.DrJanet.com: For nutrition tips, recipes, blogs, book and app links, and all things nutritious and healthy, visit my website. You can also find out about my extensive credentials so you can have full confidence in my written nutrition advice.

>> www.MediterraneanNutritionist.com: This website is your one-stop Mediterranean eating guide. *U.S. News & World Report* has consistently rated the Mediterranean Diet as No. 1 in numerous categories.

Where to Go from Here

You can read the entire book from cover to cover or if that's not how you want to go about it, feel free to go to the Table of Contents and read the chapters that most interest you right now. You may want to start in the kitchen or supermarket, stocking up on delicious, nutritious foods for recipes in Chapters 21 and 22. Perhaps you may want to start with Chapter 1 to get an overview of intermittent fasting. Or you may decide to peruse the Parts of Tens first to get a quick overview of key recommendations in bite-sized bits of information. Regardless, this journey is all about putting you in charge. It's about *you* taking control of your life and changing *when* you eat while still enabling you to choose what you eat.

If you want additional information to reference whenever you want, refer to the Cheat Sheet at www.dummies.com. Just search for "Intermittent Fasting For Dummies Cheat Sheet."

1
Getting Started with Intermittent Fasting

IN THIS PART . . .

Find out what intermittent fasting is and why this eating pattern is a complete game-changer.

Evaluate whether intermittent fasting is a lifestyle that's feasible for you and what you need to do if it is.

Assess where you're beginning so you can figure out where you want to go with your intermittent fasting plan.

Determine your ideal weight range for your personal health to get you a clearer picture of what is a safe and sustainable weight and percent body fat goal.

Get up to speed on this exciting method of losing body fat (especially the dangerous belly fat) and getting healthier.

Chapter **1**

The Lowdown on Intermittent Fasting, Just the Basics

You want to begin an intermittent fasting plan and embark on a leaner, healthier, and longer life. (You wouldn't be reading this book otherwise, right?) You may have heard that intermittent fasting is the key that unlocks everything from sustainable weight loss to increased mental clarity to a serious boost in energy. You may have asked your healthcare provider about how to follow this wildly popular diet but given her limited nutrition knowledge, you may not have received valid information.

So in vogue is this health and fitness trend, that it has moved into fad diet territory — meaning intensely popular for a short period of time — spawning massive amounts of misinformation at your fingertips. Because of its fad status, you may have fallen prey to illegitimate intermittent fasting claims and techniques proliferating on the Internet. This chapter serves as your jumping-off point to the world of intermittent fasting and explains in plain English what intermittent fasting is, based on sound science.

Defining Exactly What Intermittent Fasting Is (and Isn't)

Before you can understand what intermittent fasting is, I first need to discuss fasting, which is different from intermittent fasting. *Fasting* is refraining from consuming food or drinks, except for water, for a set period. Traditional fasting, for lengthy periods of time, isn't a healthy means of weight loss and can be extremely dangerous. In fact, long-term fasting starves the body of essential nutrients, causes the body to shut down (metabolism slows dramatically), and can be life threatening.

CLARIFYING STARVATION MODE: HINT, IT'S A MYTH

This nutrition myth pervades the dieting world, with confusion occurring because the term *starvation mode* means many different things to many different people. The often-repeated belief is that when trying to lose weight, you shouldn't drop your calories too low, because your body will go into starvation mode, and you'll hold onto fat and stop losing weight. This is 100 percent false. You don't gain weight or fat from eating too little. You won't go into a starvation mode during your intermittent fasting regimen.

Consider these facts:

- The starvation mode refers to the reduction in metabolic rate that occurs when the body is starved for long periods of time, such as observed in severely malnourished people with anorexia nervosa.

- During severe starvation, the body does in fact slow its metabolism down, dramatically; the body's natural physiological response to an extreme reduction in calorie intake, a technique the body uses as a survival mechanism. Without it, humans would have become extinct thousands of years ago.

- The starvation mode does *not* occur during most people's dieting experiences. Dieting, even low-calorie diets, don't catapult your body into starvation mode.

- When you lose weight, your body will require less calories to maintain your new body weight because there's less of you, so you require fewer calories, a concept referred to as *metabolic adaptation*.

- You can offset this metabolic adaptation and keep your metabolism as high as possible when losing weight by adding in strength-training exercise and making sure you eat enough protein.

However, *intermittent fasting* differs from traditional fasting. As the name suggests, intermittent fasting refers to alternating periods of fasting with periods of eating. It's a broad term, encompassing several specific types of short-term fasting protocols. The common theme among intermittent fasting regimens is that people periodically abstain from eating for periods longer than the typical overnight fast. Individuals either fast during a certain window every day or block out certain days of the week. These short eating rest periods allow the body's numerous systems to rest and reset without triggering the risk of malnutrition and metabolic slowdown that accompanies severely restrictive long-term fasting regimens.

Here I take a closer look at what intermittent fasting is and some of the dos and don'ts of getting started on your intermittent fasting journey.

Recognizing the nuts and bolts of intermittent fasting

Here are the key principles of intermittent fasting lifestyle methods:

>> **All intermittent fasts restrict eating and drinking for set, short periods of time.** Every method of intermittent fasting outlined in Part 3 has feasting and fasting periods that vary, depending on the regimen.

>> **The intermittent fasting approach involves alternating periods of eating and fasting.** These time periods differ depending on the variation of intermittent fasting, so you choose the method that works best for your lifestyle.

>> **All intermittent fasting protocols are safe and effective for healthy individuals.** Each of the methods in Part 3 are safe and have been shown to improve a person's health and well-being, if practiced correctly.

>> **All intermittent fasting protocols have certain rules you must follow during your fasting window.** These steps include drinking plentiful amounts of water, black coffee, tea, and any other non-caloric beverage during your fasting window; just no solid foods allowed. Make sure to stay hydrated during your intermittent fasting periods.

>> **All intermittent fasting protocols prohibit you from eating excessive amounts of junk food during your eating windows.** This habit will negate the many benefits of intermittent fasting. The biggest mistake people make is eating too much and eating unhealthy foods during their eating periods.

> » **Intermittent fasting can be practiced for health and fitness and not necessarily for weight loss.** Although weight loss is one of the most common reasons for trying intermittent fasting, many people choose to get leaner and fitter and tap into the numerous health benefits intermittent fasting provides without the goal of losing weight. In fact, some follow an intermittent fasting program with the primary goal of gaining muscle weight and losing body fat.

Although intermittent fasting is a healthy choice for some, for others, it can be dangerous. Several groups of people who absolutely *should not fast* include the following:

- » Pregnant or lactating women

- » Individuals who have eating disorders

- » Individuals with type 1 or type 2 diabetes unless working with their healthcare professional (physicians *must* be consulted if you have any underlying chronic disease)

- » Individuals using medications that they must take with food, unless working with their physician

- » High-level endurance athletes

- » Elderly individuals with balance issues

- » Children

Chapter 7 discusses in greater detail who should and shouldn't follow an intermittent fasting plan.

Delving deeper into how intermittent fasting works

Intermittent fasts cycle between periods of fasting with periods of eating. Whether or not you're fasting, the body still requires energy to run efficiently. The body's main source of energy is a sugar called *glucose,* which typically comes from carbohydrates such as grains, fruits, vegetables, and even sweets. Both your liver and muscles store the sugar and release it into the bloodstream whenever the body needs it.

Looking closer at the physiology

To understand how intermittent fasting works, you need a quick adaptive physiology refresher. Because food wasn't always abundant, and sometimes wasn't available at all, the human body was forced to adapt to fasting involuntarily — and then, when Stone Age humans found food, they would feast. Because of those evolutionary conditions, human bodies evolved to permit their bodies to thrive by adapting to those cycles of feasting and fasting. In order to survive in such environments where food was scarce, humans had to possess the ability to quickly shift their metabolism from fat storage to fat breakdown for energy. This metabolic flexibility became built into human's genetic code, producing a system where energy was stored in the form of body fat when food was available and then easily accessed for energy to enable humans to perform at a high level, physically, during extended periods when food wasn't available. This pattern enabled human brains and bodies to function optimally in a food deprived/fasted state, giving the human race a survival advantage.

Scientists have hypothesized that the human body's adaptive benefits of intermittent fasting led to the superior cognitive capabilities (brain power) of humans compared to other mammals. These brain adaptations facilitated human's ability to invent tools, novel hunting methods, animal domestication, agriculture and food storage, and processing.

Because intermittent fasting patterns can replicate the feast-or-famine diet of human ancestors, many researchers have now recognized the advantages of periodically fasting (such as increased brain power, physical enhancements, and disease prevention) for the multitude of health benefits this lifestyle gives rise to.

Examining the timeline of events

What is the physiology of fasting? Although everybody responds to fasting a little differently (genetics, health, and age all play a role), there is a general timeline of events — a predictable set of metabolic responses as your fast stretches from hours into a day or longer. (For a much more detailed discussion of the different metabolic states your body goes through when practicing intermittent fasting, refer to Chapter 5.)

REMEMBER

After fasting for a mere eight hours, here is the timeline of what happens in your body:

1. **You have no food coming in, so you exhaust your supplies.**

   Your body has tapped into your liver reserves of blood sugar to continue to keep your blood sugar level in the normal range. You're now in what's termed a *catabolic* or breakdown state.

2. **You enter the fasted state; your liver has run out of its sugar reserves.**

   This triggers the liver to manufacture new sugar from noncarbohydrate sources (scientifically termed *gluconeogenesis*) to continue to supply energy to the cells. With no carbohydrates consumed, the body creates its own sugar by using mainly fat. This marks the body's transition into the fasting mode. Studies have shown that gluconeogenesis increases the number of calories the body burns, meaning when your metabolism starts to increase.

3. You flip your metabolic switch.

One key mechanism responsible for many of the beneficial health effects of short-term, intermittent fasting is flipping of the metabolic switch. The *metabolic switch* is the body's preferential shift from utilization of blood sugar to fat and fat-derived ketones for energy. In this step, your body breaks down fat, shuttling it to the liver, which creates ketones from fat to use for energy. The metabolic switch typically occurs between 12 to 36 hours after cessation of eating.

4. Extended fasts (longer than 36 hours) begin to slow metabolism down.

That's why you shouldn't practice extended fasting with intermittent plans. After about 36 hours, the body stops using these energy sources (sugar and fat). The fasting mode then transitions to the more serious starvation mode.

5. You enter starvation mode.

At this point, your metabolism has slowed dramatically, and your body begins to burn your own muscle protein for energy. The lack of essential nutrient intake plus using muscle for energy sets off an alarming cascade of dangerous complications.

WARNING

During your recommended intermittent fasting periods, your fasting periods shouldn't extend beyond 36 hours. Although some people choose to fast for up to 48 hours, I recommend your intermittent fasting periods don't extend 36 hours because of the physiological reasons I mention here. Chapter 5 probes much deeper into the science of intermittent fasting.

Considering Your Intermittent Fasting Options

The most effective dietary plan is the one you can adhere to for the long term while still living your best life. If you want to lose weight and are sick and tired of counting calories, then this eating pattern may be the right fit for you. The popularity of intermittent fasting lies in its simplicity and the fact that the fasting periods are time-limited, which people find easier to maintain than traditional diets.

Intermittent fasting is not only for people who want to lose weight, but it's also a phenomenal lifestyle plan for individuals who want to improve their health, fight aging, and simplify their lifestyle. The scientific data shows intermittent fasting has powerful effects on your body and brain and may even extend your life. Chapter 6 discusses the miraculous health benefits linked to intermittent fasting.

Part 3 discusses the five most common ways of practicing intermittent fasting in detail. These different alternative protocols are as follows:

>> **Time-restricted intermittent fasting:** The *time-restricted intermittent fasting,* also called the *eating window plan,* is by far the most popular plan, because many rave about it being the easiest to follow. This plan consists of fasting for a daily 16-, 18-, or 20-hour consecutive period and setting your daily eating window for the remaining 8, 6, or 4 hours (albeit, you can use other time windows). Check out Chapter 9 for more details.

>> **Warrior intermittent fasting plan:** The *warrior intermittent fasting* plan is based on the eating patterns of ancient warriors who ate very little during the day and then feasted at night. Flip to Chapter 10 for the details on this method of intermittent fasting.

>> **Alternate day intermittent fasting:** *Alternate day fasting (ADF),* another form of intermittent fasting, involves fasting one day, eating the next, and repeating. Chapter 11 gives you the lowdown on this method.

>> **5:2 intermittent fasting plan:** The *5:2 plan,* also known as the *fast diet,* entails eating 500 to 600 calories on two nonconsecutive days of the week. Chapter 12 explains the ins and outs of this plan.

>> **Eat-stop-eat intermittent fasting:** This plan requires fasting for a full 24 hours, once or twice a week. Head to Chapter 13 for how to incorporate eat-stop-eat intermittent fasting into your life.

TIP

Choosing the best intermittent fasting plan is simply a matter of preference. All the intermittent fasts in this book, if followed as directed, will result in weight loss (if desired), maintenance of muscle mass, and myriad additional health benefits. My goal is to explain all of them so that *you* can choose the one that fits you best. Remember, you are the one in control. The ideal intermittent fasting method for you is the one that is most sustainable and easiest to stick with. If you try one and it doesn't help you achieve your health and wellness goals in a reasonable time frame, switch to another. In fact, switching up your fasting plan can be beneficial as well, from a physiological standpoint. You may also consider assessing some of your barriers to change by doing some of the journaling exercises suggested in Chapters 2 and 23.

MAKING THE EVOLUTION CONNECTION WITH TODAY'S INTERMITTENT FASTING

For more than a hundred thousand years, humans roamed the earth. They were foragers, so they'd fast until they found, caught, or killed their food. Like so many animals in the wild, human's paleolithic ancestors regularly experienced extended time periods with little or no food. The timing of eating depended on the availability of food; they ate opportunistically. Because humans evolved in environments where food was relatively scarce, they developed numerous adaptations that enabled them to function at a high level, both physically and cognitively, when in a food-deprived/fasted state. Importantly, metabolic, endocrine, and nervous systems evolved in ways that facilitated high levels of physical and mental performance when in the fasted state (from approximately 12 to 36 hours without food). Both the metabolic shift to ketone utilization (a chemical derivative of fat), and adaptive responses of the brain and nervous system to food deprivation play major roles in the fitness-promoting and disease-allaying effects of intermittent fasting.

Hunter-gatherers gathered berries off bushes; dug up tubers; hunted mammals; scavenged meat, fat, and organs from previously killed carcasses; and discovered how to fish and hunt with spears, nets, bows, and arrows. Furthermore, their activity level is a far cry from the sedentary lifestyle so many people today lead. By the 20th century, most hunter-gatherers had vanished from the face of the earth (currently only a few scattered tribes of hunter-gatherers remain on the planet).

Then came farming

Some 10,000 to 12,000 years ago, things began to change. Homo sapiens altered their lifestyle from hunting and gathering to a more sedentary routine of farming — what's termed the *agricultural revolution*. The human diet also took a major turn with the invention of agriculture. The domestication of grains created a plentiful and predictable food supply — *food security* — which allowed for storing surplus food. Provisions became readily available, hence people no longer had to eat opportunistically, and fasting was no longer necessary. The development of agriculture also brought a great societal transformation. People shifted from a nomadic existence to living in permanent communities, agrarian cultures.

The Industrial Revolution changed it all

Then the Industrial Revolution happened in the United States from the mid-19th century until the early 20th century. This shift in work routines permanently altered the way Americans eat. Refrigeration and transportation allowed for storing, packaging, and transporting of foods. Work shifted from farm to factory, and the human-eating schedule went to the three-meals-per-day routine that is the current eating pattern. Today, most Americans eat three meals and multiple snacks and rarely go more than four daytime hours without eating.

Answering Your Frequently Asked Questions

Intermittent fasting is right for anyone seeking a longer, healthier life. However, as a new phenomenon, you may have a host of questions that you want answered to help you determine whether intermittent fasting is right for you. Here are some common questions and answers to help you make that decision:

>> **Is hunger hard to deal with when practicing intermittent fasting?** In the beginning, you'll feel hunger pangs during your fasting periods. Most intermittent fasting newbies figure out how to accept, adjust, and dull hunger pangs, which typically dissipate after about a month on an intermittent fasting program. I explore how you can deal with the potential negative side effects of intermittent fasting in depth in Chapter 15.

>> **Do you have to exercise when practicing intermittent fasting?** Yes, but no marathons are required! All Americans need to move more for better health. Because you're entering into a lifestyle program aimed at improving your health, this one does indeed advocate daily exercise. Chapter 14 explores the specifics on exercise.

>> **How long should you fast for?** You'll see health benefits from fasts of from 14 hours to 36 hours. The ideal fasting window and ultimately fasting regimen will vary depending on you. What matters is the duration of fasting that works for your lifestyle.

>> **Can you drink alcohol when practicing intermittent fasting?** Yes, you can during your eating windows, in moderation, and if you can drink responsibly. You should know that drinking any amount of alcohol increases your risk of seven different types of cancer.

>> **Can you have a cheat day during intermittent fasting?** One of the phenomenal attractions of intermittent fasting is the concept that you get lots of cheat days — built in. Technically, you can eat whatever you want during your eating windows. This simple idea of freedom in eating is very motivating — fast today for tomorrow you feast!

>> **Can you gain muscle when practicing intermittent fasting?** Yes, studies have shown that combining intermittent fasting with a program of strength-training designed to increase muscle mass will result in muscle gain and fat loss. For details on how to gain muscle while practicing intermittent fasting, flip to Chapter 14.

WHAT DID THE CAVEMAN REALLY EAT? THINK OINK, OINK

Well, it sure wasn't filet mignon! Human ancestors evolved as hunters and gatherers; for hundreds of thousands of years, their lives were spent searching for food. Believe it or not, some scientists believe that *early humans had a diet like pigs*. (Pigs are *omnivores*, meaning they consume both plants and animals. In the wild, they forage for anything and everything edible such as leaves, roots, fruits, flowers, insects, and fish.) What can be said for certain is that in the Paleolithic age, the human diet varied immensely by geography, season, and opportunity. Humans were flexible eaters, opportunistic eaters who ate what was available depending on their geographic locale. For example, humans in the Arctic ate almost all animal foods (seafood), whereas populations in the Andes sustained themselves on primarily plant foods (tubers and cereal grains).

>> **Can you take medications and supplements when practicing intermittent fasting?** Yes, you must continue taking your prescription medications as directed (and should only practice intermittent fasting under the guidance of your personal healthcare provider). If you need to take your meds with food, on a daily basis, choose an intermittent fasting plan that allows a daily window of eating for your medications. Supplements, as long as they contain negligible calories, can be taken as usual. Check with your healthcare provider if you have any concerns.

Taking the First Steps of Change

Intermittent fasting is a major lifestyle change for everyone. Before you commit to taking the first steps or just diving right in, you may be interested in discovering the basic steps of making major life changes. The three basic steps for change are:

1. **Know yourself.**

After you do that, you can grasp what you need to change and be able to gauge how much you've changed. You'll be figuring how to take a personal inventory and how to set SMART goals that I discuss in Chapter 2. Take baby steps and focus on achieving small goals every day.

2. **Take away the knowledge in this book as power.**

   Find the wisdom that for you is most relevant and leave behind the rest of the words that don't help you.

3. **Practice what you've read.**

   Imbibe the principles and carry them out in your life. Fight back against procrastination and inactivity and vigorously apply the knowledge you have acquired.

Life is complicated, and intermittent fasting simplifies it. Food is expensive; with intermittent fasting, you save money. Shopping, cooking, and cleaning up meals is time consuming; intermittent fasting saves you time. These benefits are what make intermittent fasting so popular among the life hacker crowd. Life hacks are strategies or techniques adopted to manage one's time and daily activities in a more efficient way. Adopting life hacks is all about eliminating life's manifold frustrations in simple and ingenious ways. Take your first steps of change by hopping on the intermittent fasting bandwagon and start today to sooth your brain by mitigating some of life's stress.

Chapter **2**

Assessing Your Goals

N o lifestyle change program will work until you set a goal for success. Achievable goals serve as your road map markers for your entire lifestyle-change journey. Without these guides, you're like a driver who hops in the car and starts driving without any idea of where he or she's going.

But before you figure out how to set your goals, you need to begin by taking an honest self-inventory — a process that will toughen your resolve and help you succeed in your intermittent fasting lifestyle. With that information, you can summon the strength to keep taking steps forward and overcome the occasional roadblocks that life inevitably sends our way.

Having a firm grasp of your current weight and body composition is also very valuable information. Knowing where you are when you start can help you to track your progress as you incorporate intermittent fasting into your lifestyle.

This chapter is all about assessing where you are now and establishing where you want to go (your long-term health and fitness goals). Following one of the intermittent fasting plans that I discuss in Part 3 can give you what you need to achieve your goals and stay healthy and fit for life.

Understanding What a Healthy Weight Range Is for You

If you want to lose weight from intermittent fasting, you first need to know what a healthy weight range is for you. With that information, you can better understand what your short-terms goals are (baby steps) and your long-term goals or healthy weight range (your finish line).

REMEMBER

The benefits of losing weight aren't just cosmetic. Getting to a healthy weight can remediate and prevent dangerous health conditions that contribute to a shorter life. You also get a self-esteem boost, another valuable benefit.

You may be okay with your current weight and simply want to hop on the intermittent fasting train for the additional health benefits derived from this eating pattern such as disease prevention and anti-aging effects. If so, feel free to skip to Part 3 and dive right into an intermittent fasting plan that is right for you.

WARNING

If you're considering intermittent fasting, make sure you first consult your doctor. Intermittent fasting must be conducted under the watchful eye of your personal doctor if you have been previously diagnosed with a chronic disease. If you have an eating disorder, intermittent fasting absolutely isn't allowed.

People come in all sizes and shapes, with different life experiences related to their personal health and fitness. Before you estimate what a healthy weight range is for you, you need to take several preliminary steps to help you get a clearer picture of what healthy weight range is right for you.

Taking a self-inventory

A fearless self-inventory and your weight history help you get to the root of your battle of the bulge. With this information, you can cut through past experiences and grasp the power that food has had over your life. If knowledge is power, then knowing yourself better helps you gain power over your eating habits.

The questions in this self-inventory also can help you realize that you can't change history — but you can equip and strengthen yourself for the future. Look closely and honestly at your past efforts, challenges, and previous weight-loss success. Defining why you want to lose weight may help you stay motivated when complacency sets in.

Put yourself under a microscope and ask yourself these questions. Jot down your responses in your journal or notebook (refer to Chapter 23 for more about journaling your intermittent fasting voyage).

>> Were you overweight as a child? If so, how did your parent(s) react?

>> Does your weight affect your self-esteem? If yes, describe how.

>> Does your weight or the scale number affect your mood? If yes, describe how.

>> Does your weight affect your relationships? If yes, describe how.

>> Do you reach for comfort food in times of stress? If yes, describe how and when.

>> Does fitting into clothes or not fitting into them affect your mood? If yes, describe how.

>> How many diets have you tried in your lifetime? Describe them.

>> If you lost weight in the past, were you able to keep it off? If yes, how?

>> If you lost weight in the past and gained it back, what were the circumstances?

>> If you overeat or binge eat, what triggers that behavior and what time of day does it occur?

>> What is the lowest weight that you have been able to maintain as an adult for at least several months? What were the circumstances?

>> When you were at a weight in your adult life that you were happy with? What was your activity level? What were the circumstances?

>> Has your doctor ever expressed concern about your weight? If yes, describe her conversation with you.

This inventory can help you be empowered to change your life. I encourage you to revisit your answers periodically during your intermittent fasting journey. Reading your life history as it pertains to your weight can be a powerful motivator to get you back on track, should an obstacle arise in your newfound lifestyle.

Considering your reasons for weight loss

Following a reduced calorie healthy diet and exercise plan can unquestionably help you lose weight. Analyzing the reasons that drive you to lose the weight in the first place will aid you in your efforts to keep weight off. Being introspective about the real reason you want to lose weight facilitates your success in achieving your goals and is a powerful motivator for acting on and maintaining your goals.

Here are many of the most common reasons people want to lose weight. Figure out which ones motivate you the most:

» **Maintaining good health:** Being overweight is bad for your health; it raises blood pressure (the silent killer) and increases risk of heart disease, diabetes, and certain types of cancers (such as breast cancer). Avoiding these diseases can be a strong motivator for people to want to lose weight. Living a healthy lifestyle leads to living a longer and higher quality of life.

» **Boosting your energy level:** This reason may seem counterintuitive, but intermittent fasting leads to an energy boost. Extra body fat requires energy to maintain, so lose the fat and you redirect all that energy to living life.

» **Feeling better about oneself:** Society denigrates the overweight with a barrage of messages that thin is in and fat is ugly. This very real social shaming can take a toll on peoples' self-esteem. Embarrassment about one's looks can diminish self-confidence, which can lead to anxiety and depression. Feeling better about oneself and looking good is a compelling incentive to shed those pounds.

» **Decreasing joint problems:** One of the common side effects of excess body weight is joint pain, especially in the knees. Too much body weight stresses the joints and can lead to wear and tear, potentially resulting in arthritis. Joint pain can be extraordinarily painful, which creates a viscous circle, increasing weight gain by curtailing the ability to exercise.

Setting your weekly SMART goals

When choosing to follow a new lifestyle, you'll need to change behaviors. Behavior change requires determination and practice, but most of all, you need to know how to set goals that work for you that are achievable. Lasting behavior change relies on goal setting. Ideally, you want to set one small goal every week. To give you the best chance of success, your goals should:

» Represent concrete actions and not wishful thinking

» Incorporate your own personal preferences and activities that you enjoy, which will increase the likelihood of attaining your goals

» Be written in the form of SMART goals

These sections examine in greater detail what SMART goals are and how you can form your own goals.

Understanding what SMART goals are

A SMART goal is created with the following in mind:

>> **Specific:** Say exactly what you want to achieve such as "I'll confine my eating window to a specified eight-hour window, every day for the next seven days," instead of "I want to follow the 16:8 intermittent fasting plan."

>> **Measurable:** You need to be able to verify that you attained your goal. For example, "I'll mark off on my intermittent fasting schedule that I ate during my set fasting window every day," instead of "I'll choose what time I want to eat, each day as it comes."

>> **Actionable:** Meaning your goal is action oriented. "I'll eat between the hours of 12 p.m. and 8 p.m., every day and only drink calorie-free beverages during my fasting hours." Eating and drinking are action verbs.

>> **Realistic:** Your goal should be something you believe you can achieve, not something too difficult. If you know with 100 percent certainty that you can easily avoid eating or drinking calorie-containing foods from the time you wake up until 1 p.m. and continue fasting from 8 p.m. until noon the next day, then this goal is realistic for you.

>> **Time-bound:** Setting a deadline for your goal is important, so you have an end in sight. One week is a doable time frame for most people. If you plan to follow the 16:8 intermittent fast, map out a one-week schedule in advance — it's motivating because it gives you a set, doable, time frame.

Forming your own SMART goals

Use your answers to the questions in the previous section to formulate your SMART goal. For example, "This week, I'll walk 20 minutes on my treadmill, every day at 3 p.m. for the next 7 days, at a 20–minute per mile pace." This is a SMART goal instead of "I want to start an exercise program." Look at how this goal is broken down:

>> **Specific:** Walking on the treadmill for 20 minutes is specific.

>> **Measurable:** You measure 20 minutes on the treadmill.

>> **Actionable:** Walking is an action.

>> **Realistic:** This plan of action is doable if you've previously walked for exercise.

>> **Time-bound**: Walking for 20 minutes for the next 7 days is time-related.

TIP

Write your first weekly SMART goal in a journal of your choice, on your smart phone memo pad, or on a sheet of paper that you copied from Chapter 23. Make your goal something small, one that you're 100 percent positive that you'll accomplish.

After you've finished your first weekly SMART goal, you're not done. Ask yourself the following:

>> Did I achieve my goal this week?

>> If yes, then take the time to create a new one.

>> If no, then analyze where the problem was and then create a new, more achievable goal.

TIP

In addition to your significant small, weekly SMART goal, you can set a big-picture, long-term goal. Setting long-term goals of, say three months, is helpful for mapping out your intermittent fasting journey. Three months is like goldilocks — not too far off, but still close enough to be palpable. Your long-term goal sheet will cover not only weight goals but also health and fitness goals. You can find a blank three-month weight, health and fitness goal sheet in Chapter 23.

Here is an example of a realistic three-month goal:

Weight: I'll lose 10 pounds in the next three months. I'll measure my weight on the scale to track my progress.

Health: Losing this weight will help lower my blood sugar (I am pre-diabetic) to reduce my risk for diabetes. I'll test my fasting blood sugar to track this health marker.

Fitness: Losing fat and becoming a fitter person will help me to move more comfortably when I go hiking with my kids. I'll test this by completing the one-mile hike that I currently cannot finish.

Taking action after you reach your goals

If you don't reach your weekly goal, no big deal, just formulate a new weekly SMART goal. Ensure that this week's SMART goal is going to be more achievable. If you did achieve your goal, reward yourself — no need for anything expensive — a simple pleasure such as buying a new book, getting a massage, or soaking in a hot bath, whatever makes you happy.

After you achieve your long-term goals, have a big celebration! You can pencil into your calendar something that's really important for you to reward yourself with and cross off those days and weeks as you get closer and closer to that day.

Calculating Your Healthy Weight Range

Nutritionists use several different tools to calculate a person's healthy weight range. The good news, you don't need to be an expert to use many of those same assessments.

REMEMBER

The following sections examine many of these different ways you can calculate your healthy weight and what you can then do with those numbers. Defining how you measure your success as you move through your journey is extremely important. For example, you may choose to utilize one of the following tools, whereas other people may choose another. No matter which one or ones you choose, each is a different way to measure changes to your body's size. After you decide, be specific about which measurement or multiple measurements you use to stay accountable to your goals and track them using your journaling technique of choice. Ultimately, a healthy weight *for you* is the weight range that can help you prevent and/or manage chronic disease.

Making friends with the scale

Scientists concur that keeping tabs on your progress by weighing yourself often (and recording the weight) is one of the best tools for helping you achieve your weight-loss goals. In fact, stepping on the scale is the best way to assess whether your intermittent fasting program is working for you. If you don't see a drop in weight over time, then you need to reassess your program and tweak your plan. If you're trying to hit a specific number or weight range, weighing yourself is the simplest and most accurate means of determining your starting point and whether you've reached your goal.

You may hate the idea of the scale, but frequent self-weighing is not only beneficial for losing weight, but it also helps prevent weight gain associated with aging as well as stopping weight regain after loss. Be brave, step on that scale!

REMEMBER

Keep the following pointers in mind as you weigh yourself to ensure your results are as accurate as possible:

>> **Remember not all scales are created equally.** Different scales can yield different results at different times of day. Therefore, experts recommend routinely using the same scale to highlight your progress.

>> **Weigh in the morning.** If you weigh yourself at night, especially after you've eaten, you're going to weigh more than you truly do. Weigh yourself first thing in the morning, unclothed, and definitely *not* after an exercise bout.

>> **Wear your birthday suit.** Clothes can add up to two pounds on the scale that don't account for your actual body weight. Weigh yourself unclothed.

>> **Don't weigh every day.** You won't see major changes from day to day and checking the scale that frequently can do more harm than good by affecting your mood and motivation. Twice a week is ideal.

>> **You don't take a holistic approach.** The number on the scale shouldn't be the only measure of your success. Just because the numbers on the scale aren't moving, or aren't moving fast enough for you, doesn't mean your body isn't changing in a positive direction. You can still be losing fat, perhaps gaining a tad of muscle, and looking at your newfound energy boost as positive markers that your healthy lifestyle is working.

When you're trying to lose weight, you can easily let the number on the scale ruin your day. Don't overstress it. You may have eaten too much water- retaining sodium, you may be adding muscle, or you may have overeaten. Weight fluctuates naturally, and because weight on a scale isn't always reflective of other positive changes that are happening in your body, I suggest you use other methods of assessment tools that I outline in the following sections.

REMEMBER

Weighing yourself is *not* mandatory when following an intermittent fasting program. You're weighing yourself to obtain data, not to judge yourself. However, if the scale isn't an assessment tool you want to use, then ditch it!

Guesstimating accurately

Starting with a rough idea of your healthy weight is better than nothing. Here's a quick, down and dirty calculation that can give you a fast estimate of whether you're overweight. Since this calculation was originally created, many nations' populations have literally expanded and people have gotten heavier. Therefore, keep in mind, that this guesstimate tends to make your ideal weight range much lower compared to the other calculations in this chapter:

>> **For men:** Start with 106 pounds for 5 feet in height and then add 6 pounds per inch where you're taller than 5 feet or subtract 6 pounds per inch if you're shorter than 5 feet. The healthy weight range would be plus or minus 10 percent.

>> **For women:** Start with 100 pounds for 5 feet in height and then add 5 pounds per inch where you're taller than 5 feet or subtract 5 pounds per inch if you're shorter than 5 feet. The healthy weight range would be plus or minus 10 percent.

WARNING

All the calculations and assessments in this chapter are for adults only. Children should be assessed by their pediatrician or a pediatric dietitian.

Here's an example of this method:

> Debbie is a 50-year-old woman. She is 5-5 tall and weighs 160 pounds.
>
> Her healthy weight range would be $\{100 + (5 \times 5)\} =$
>
> $$125 \text{ pounds } (125 \times .10 = 12.5 \text{ pounds}\}$$
>
> $$\{125 + 12.5 = 137.5\}$$
> $$\{125 - 12.5 = 112.5\}$$

Debbie's healthy weight range is between 112.5 pounds and 137.5 pounds. Therefore, according to this method (which does tend to underestimate ideal weight range), Debbie needs to lose approximately 20 pounds to reach her healthy weight goal.

WEB EXTRAS

You can access one of my favorite websites (`www.calculator.net/ideal-weight-calculator.html`) that uses several popular science-based weight formulas (based on your height, gender, and age) and then displays the results side-by-side to allow you to see your ideal weight at the click of your mouse. Plugging Debbie's age and height into the calculator gives you a range of ideal body weights from 125 to 132 pounds.

Using your Body Mass Index to see whether you're overweight

Doctors use a mass screening tool to give them another quick way to instantly see if their patient's weight puts their patient at risk for health problems. The *body mass index (BMI)* is a good estimate of body fat, based on height and weight, that applies only to adult men and women.

The National Institutes of Health (NIH) defines BMI categories as such:

>> **Healthy weight:** 18.5 to 24.9

>> **Overweight:** 25 to 29.9

>> **Obese:** 30 or greater

REMEMBER

You want to aim for a healthy BMI of *less than 25*. Figure 2-1 shows a BMI chart where you can look up your BMI.

WEB EXTRAS

The National Institutes of Health (NIH) has a great BMI calculator at `www.nhlbi.nih.gov/health/educational/lose_wt/BMI/bmicalc.htm` that does the work for you.

Body Mass Index Table

Category spans: Normal (BMI 19–24) · Overweight (BMI 25–29) · Obese (BMI 30–39) · Extreme Obesity (BMI 40–54)

Body Weight (pounds)

BMI / Height (inches)	19	20	21	22	23	24	25	26	27	28	29	30	31	32	33	34	35	36	37	38	39	40	41	42	43	44	45	46	47	48	49	50	51	52	53	54
58	91	96	100	105	110	115	119	124	129	134	138	143	148	153	158	162	167	172	177	181	186	191	196	201	205	210	215	220	224	229	234	239	244	248	253	258
59	94	99	104	109	114	119	124	128	133	138	143	148	153	158	163	168	173	178	183	188	193	198	203	208	212	217	222	227	232	237	242	247	252	257	262	267
60	97	102	107	112	118	123	128	133	138	143	148	153	158	163	168	174	179	184	189	194	199	204	209	215	220	225	230	235	240	245	250	255	261	266	271	276
61	100	106	111	116	122	127	132	137	143	148	153	158	164	169	174	180	185	190	195	201	206	211	217	222	227	232	238	243	248	254	259	264	269	275	280	285
62	104	109	115	120	126	131	136	142	147	153	158	164	169	175	180	186	191	196	202	207	213	218	224	229	235	240	246	251	256	262	267	273	278	284	289	295
63	107	113	118	124	130	135	141	146	152	158	163	169	175	180	186	191	197	203	208	214	220	225	231	237	242	248	254	259	265	270	278	282	287	293	299	304
64	110	116	122	128	134	140	145	151	157	163	169	174	180	186	192	197	204	209	215	221	227	232	238	244	250	256	262	267	273	279	285	291	296	302	308	314
65	114	120	126	132	138	144	150	156	162	168	174	180	186	192	198	204	210	216	222	228	234	240	246	252	258	264	270	276	282	288	294	300	306	312	318	324
66	118	124	130	136	142	148	155	161	167	173	179	186	192	198	204	210	216	223	229	235	241	247	253	260	266	272	278	284	291	297	303	309	315	322	328	334
67	121	127	134	140	146	153	159	166	172	178	185	191	198	204	211	217	223	230	236	242	249	255	261	268	274	280	287	293	299	306	312	319	325	331	338	344
68	125	131	138	144	151	158	164	171	177	184	190	197	203	210	216	223	230	236	243	249	256	262	269	276	282	289	295	302	308	315	322	328	335	341	348	354
69	128	135	142	149	155	162	169	176	182	189	196	203	209	216	223	230	236	243	250	257	263	270	277	284	291	297	304	311	318	324	331	338	345	351	358	365
70	132	139	146	153	160	167	174	181	188	195	202	209	216	222	229	236	243	250	257	264	271	278	285	292	299	306	313	320	327	334	341	348	355	362	369	376
71	136	143	150	157	165	172	179	186	193	200	208	215	222	229	236	243	250	257	265	272	279	286	293	301	308	315	322	329	338	343	351	358	365	372	379	386
72	140	147	154	162	169	177	184	191	199	206	213	221	228	235	242	250	258	265	272	279	287	294	302	309	316	324	331	338	346	353	361	368	375	383	390	397
73	144	151	159	166	174	182	189	197	204	212	219	227	235	242	250	257	265	272	280	288	295	302	310	318	325	333	340	348	355	363	371	378	386	393	401	408
74	148	155	163	171	179	186	194	202	210	218	225	233	241	249	256	264	272	280	287	295	303	311	319	326	334	342	350	358	365	373	381	389	396	404	412	420
75	152	160	168	176	184	192	200	208	216	224	232	240	248	256	264	272	279	287	295	303	311	319	327	335	343	351	359	367	375	383	391	399	407	415	423	431
76	156	164	172	180	189	197	205	213	221	230	238	246	254	263	271	279	287	295	304	312	320	328	336	344	353	361	369	377	385	394	402	410	418	426	435	443

Source: Adapted from Clinical Guidelines on the Identification, Evaluation, and Treatment of Overweight and Obesity in Adults: The Evidence Report.

FIGURE 2-1: Body Mass Index chart.

Source: www.nhlbi.nih.gov/health/educational/lose_wt/BMI/bmi_tbl.pdf

If you like numbers and want to do the calculations yourself, then use this equation:

$$\text{BMI} = \left\{ \text{body weight} \left(\text{pounds} \right) \times 704.5 \right\} \div \left\{ \text{height} \left(\text{inches} \right) \times \text{height} \left(\text{inches} \right) \right\}$$

Here's how this equation works:

Use Debbie from the previous section. If you input her height and weight into the online BMI calculator, you come up with a BMI of 26.6, a number greater than 25, so Debbie is overweight. How much weight would Debbie have to lose to get to a BMI of 25? For her height she'd need to weigh a little less than 150 to get to a BMI of 25, so in this case she would set a long-term weight loss goal of 11 pounds. I suggest you use this method for an accurate calculation when you're setting your initial weight-loss goals.

WARNING

A healthy and safe rate of weight loss that virtually guarantees you're losing almost all body fat and not precious muscle mass is a maximum of 1 to 2 pounds per week. Furthermore, experts have shown that people who lose weight gradually and steadily are more successful at keeping weight from returning.

However, the BMI calculation does have its limitations, which include the following:

>> It may overestimate body fat in athletes and others who have a muscular build.

>> It can underestimate body fat in older persons and others who have lost muscle.

Gauging your inches to link your weight and health

You can use a tape measure to measure the circumference of different sites of your body as another monitor of change. When using this tool, make sure the measuring tape is around your waist because when it comes to your weight affecting your health, it may not be how much fat you have but where the fat is stored.

Most people store body fat in one of two distinct patterns:

>> **Apple shape:** Having an apple shape (extra weight carried around the stomach, often referred to as *extra belly fat*) is associated with a greater risk of developing chronic diseases such as diabetes and heart disease.

>> **Pear shape:** Having a pear shape means you carry most of your extra weight in your hips, upper thighs, and buttocks. Pear-shaped people are significantly healthier than those people with apple-shaped bodies. Fat deposited on the hips is less likely to travel around the body, reducing the risk of diabetes and heart disease.

A waist circumference measurement is a simple screening technique to determine what your shape is. If you fall into this increased health risk category (unhealthy BMI and an apple shape), then following an intermittent fasting plan is a wonderful way to help you lose that stubborn belly fat.

WARNING

The following waist measurements are red flags, suggesting that you carry fat around the abdominal area:

>> **Women 18 and older:** Waist of 35 inches or more

>> **Men 18 and older:** Waist of 40 inches or more

TIP

Follow these steps to accurately measure your waist with a tape measure:

1. **Relax and stand.**

   With a tape measure, start at the top of your hip bone and then bring the tape measure all the way around your body, raising the tape until it's at a level slightly above your belly button.

2. **Make sure the tape isn't too tight and that it's straight, even on your back.**

   Don't hold your breath while measuring because doing so can affect the results.

WARNING

3. **Check the number on the tape measure right after you exhale.**

   When you place the tape over the skin, do so just to make contact but don't compress the skin in any way.

4. **Take all measurements twice and average them.**

   Taking the measurements twice, consecutively, and then averaging the results ensures greater accuracy.

5. **Record to the nearest half-inch.**

You can repeat this measurement every few months and record the number in your journal. Tracking all your numbers in your journal, over time, gives you a motivation-boosting visual and a reward for all your hard work.

Determining what a healthy percentage of body fat is for you

Weight alone isn't a clear indicator of your health because it doesn't distinguish between pounds that come from body fat and those that come from muscle. Excess body fat is the culprit when promoting disease, so knowing what your percentage of body fat is important. The most reliable method of figuring out how much fat is in your body is to use measurements of body composition.

You can refer to professionals to measure your body fat or you can do it yourself. The following two sections examine these options in greater detail.

Seeking pros to measure your body composition

You can get reasonably accurate results from fitness centers or universities where specially trained fitness professionals use valid tools ranging from simple measurements to expensive tests to measure your body fat. Some of these techniques include skin fold calipers, underwater weighing tanks, air displacement plethysmography (Bod Pods), and bioelectrical impedance analysis (BIA) equipment.

REMEMBER

If you try several of these methods, you may receive different measurements. You basically get what you pay for. Obtaining an estimate of your body fat from unscientific methods (such as scales and untrained fitness professionals) produces notoriously erroneous results. Underwater weighing, magnetic resonance imaging, computerized tomography (CT) scans, and air displacement plethysmography are the most accurate, but they're also the costliest, unless insurance covers them. If you're able to use more than one tool, be sure to keep track of changes in your body fat over time in your journal to keep you motivated.

Some people think that the lower the amount of fat in the body, the better. However, that's not true, because the body needs a minimum percentage of fat, called *essential fat* that is lower in men (3 percent) and greater for women (12 to 15 percent) for good health. (Only elite athletes ever come close to these extremely low body fat numbers.)

Doing it yourself

You can also estimate your percent body fat yourself using a tape measure. Just follow these easy steps to get your percent body fat estimate:

1. **Measure the circumference of your waist (at the narrowest point), hips (at the widest point) and neck (at the narrowest point).**

2. Take the measurements twice and follow the same guidelines that I discuss in the "Gauging your inches to link your weight and health" for measuring your waist.

3. To calculate your body fat percentage, go to the online calculator (http://fitness.bizcalcs.com/Calculator.asp?Calc=Body-Fat-Navy), enter your gender, weight, height, and your measurements.

Voila. Your percent body fat estimate.

Here is an example using Debbie from the earlier "Guesstimating accurately" section:

Debbie is a female, weighs 150 pounds, and is 5-5. Her waist is 35 inches, her hips measure 38 inches, and her neck is 12 inches. According to the U.S. Navy formula, her body fat percentage is 36 percent. By referring to Figure 2-2 and using her age (50), you can see that Debbie's body fat percentage puts her in the overweight range — meaning her weight could put her at risk for numerous health problems.

If you determine that you're not happy with the category you're in, then you can use that info as another means to motivate yourself to exercise and stick to your intermittent fasting plan.

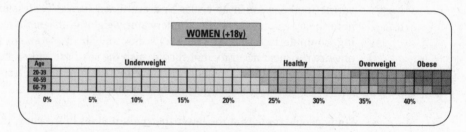

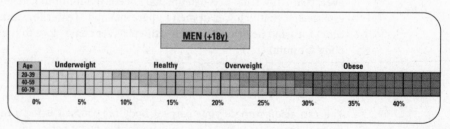

© John Wiley & Sons, Inc.

FIGURE 2-2: Percent body fat categories.

Chapter **3**

Verifying Calories As Your Last Resort

C alories . . . you hate them, you don't want to hear about them, and you certainly don't want to count them. You may even be a bit taken aback by a discussion of calories when you thought intermittent fasting didn't count calories. After all, intermittent fasting is about when you eat, not so much about what you eat, right? Yes and no. The beauty and simplicity of intermittent fasting plans lie in the focus more on timing rather than the nuisance of counting calories.

It's up to you: You can immediately skip this chapter, or you can instead use this chapter as your backup tool kit to refer to if your intermittent fasting plan is not giving you the results that you had hoped for. Or, perhaps, you're just interested in calories.

This chapter is a tool to help you grasp the concept of weight loss and the role calories play in losing and gaining weight. If one of your intermittent fasting goals is to lose weight and body fat, then the following illustrates why intermittent fasting works.

Examining How Your Intermittent Fasting Plan Is Going

People who try intermittent fasting and fail, lament that it doesn't work. The overwhelming reason *why* intermittent fasting doesn't give results for these people is because they use their fasting windows as a license to eat anything and everything they want. Bottom line: They eat too many calories during their eating windows, an action that will prevent weight loss and perhaps even promote weight gain. If you find yourself in the same situation, then press your panic button and do the calorie calculations in this chapter to see what and where you're overeating and/or underexercising. What I can tell you from my years of experience helping people lose weight is that 99.9 percent of people underestimate the amount of food they eat.

TIP

Intermittent fasting isn't a diet, but a pattern of eating. More specifically, it's a lifestyle that you can sustain for a lifetime. The key to not feeling deprived is to think of it as a marathon, not a sprint. Familiarizing yourself with the calorie math can help you to instinctively recognize when you're overeating without getting out a calculator.

Never fear! I don't advise counting your calories each day, each week, or each month. I do encourage you to do the occasional calorie calculations to make yourself more aware of what you're eating. Knowing this information can help you make better choices around food and meal selection during your eating windows as well as help you reach your weight and fat loss goals.

The next few sections take you on a whirlwind science exploration tour — the laws of physics (simplified). The goal is to clarify the misinformation that you may have been bombarded with regarding the basis for all things weight related (both weight gain and weight loss).

Explaining calorie surplus and deficit

Search for "calories and weight loss" online, and you'll find: "Not all calories are equivalent. "A calorie may not be a calorie." "A calorie is of course a calorie." As you can see, a lot of information is out there about the role calories play in weight loss.

LOOKING TO PHYSICS TO EXPLAIN CALORIES

In an effort to clarify the calorie science, this calls for a refresher on Sir Isaac Newton's laws of physics to help you understand calorie deficit. Newton's first law of thermodynamics (in physics) is the law of conservation of energy. This states that energy can't be created or destroyed in a closed system. *Translation:* If the calories in the foods you consume (even those foods you may consider to be clean) are more than the calories you burn (your resting metabolic rate and all your activity in a day), you're creating a daily calorie surplus and you're going to gain weight (fat). Simple. What about the other way around? If you eat fewer calories than you expend and create a daily calorie deficit, you'll lose weight.

The following two terms are important when talking about calories and weight loss:

>> **Calorie surplus:** You eat more calories than you expend and create a daily *calorie surplus,* you gain weight.

>> **Calorie deficit:** You eat fewer calories than you expend and create a daily *calorie deficit,* you lose weight.

All diets — regardless of macronutrient (carbs, fat, and protein) percentage (low-carb, low-fat, Paleo, vegan, Mediterranean, or even intermittent fasting plans) — work through creating a calorie deficit. If you don't create a calorie deficit, you don't lose weight. If you create too great a calorie deficit, you lose muscle mass and your metabolic rate drops (yikes!).

It's a balancing act, create the deficit, just not too much. Anyone who argues against the fundamental role of energy balance in weight regulation — against calories in versus calories out — is practicing an exercise in futility.

Even though it's a fact that calories in versus calories out is the law, it's equally true that the number of calories required to lose weight or maintain weight or gain weight differs from person to person. That's because the calories required for each person vary widely and are influenced by numerous factors not under a person's control such as genetics.

What's also true is not all calories are created equally. There is a difference in the number of calories your body requires to burn and digest each of the three macronutrients: protein, carbs, and fat —scientifically termed the *thermic effect of food.* Protein has the highest thermic effect of the three macronutrients, but the increase in metabolic rate from eating protein (and therefore its contribution to weight loss) is negligible. The great thing about eating protein when intermittent fasting is that protein is the most filling of the macronutrients. Eating protein helps curb your appetite — a welcome addition to any weight-loss plan.

Forget the marketing hype and fad diet gimmicks. When it comes to losing weight, eat fewer calories and burn more calories, and over time you *will* lose weight.

Studying Calories 101

When you cut down on your intake of one macronutrient (whether it's carbs or fat — both popular fad diet strategies), or you restrict yourself from eating for 16 hours in a particular day (such as the 16:8 intermittent fasting plan), your total calories consumed for that day will be lower than what you would have eaten on a typical day in your pre-fasting life. This action creates a calorie deficit — the all-important basis for weight loss.

A calorie isn't something tangible, like something you pick up when you hold a chocolate chip cookie. A *calorie* is instead simply a measurement also known as a unit of energy. Think of an inch as a measurement of length and a calorie as a measurement of energy.

Science has two forms of calories:

» **Calorie with a small c as in calorie:** The scientific description of a calorie is the amount of heat needed to raise the temperature of one gram of water by one degree Celsius. This calorie isn't the same one most people think of when discussing food, so I don't discuss it any further.

» **Calorie with a big C as in Calorie:** In nutritionist language it's called a *kilocalorie* or *kcal* for short. Nutritionists use these terms to refer to calories in food or to calories burned during exercise. The scientific definition of *kilocalories* is the amount of heat needed to raise the temperature of 1 kilogram of water by 1 degree Celsius. You use this calorie when reading the food labels in the supermarket. Note: Books about weight loss and weight gain refer to this type of calorie.

Balancing your equation

The energy balance equation illustrates how weight loss and gain relate to calories. In order to maintain your current weight, you need to consume approximately the same number of calories as you burn:

Calories in = Calories out

Conversely, if you want to lose weight, you need to consume fewer calories or burn more calories. For most people, a calorie deficit of 500 calories per day is just enough to promote weight and fat loss and unlikely to significantly affect your muscle mass or energy levels.

In addition to intermittent fasting, you should also increase your physical activity — to widen the calorie deficit. Intermittent fasting creates a calorie deficit through its focus on diet rather than exercise alone, a method that many find easier than attempting to lose weight through just exercise. As a general rule, weight loss is generally 75 percent diet and 25 percent exercise. However, don't nix the exercise in your intermittent fasting lifestyle because physical activity is also important for promoting better health.

Keep in mind that more muscular bodies need more calories to sustain themselves than less lean bodies. If you wish to gain weight (muscle) and still reap the rewards of intermittent fasting, then calories in should be greater than calories out. You can accomplish this by having a highly nutritious caloric-dense diet combined with a solid strength training program (refer to Chapter 14 for more about incorporating exercise into your lifestyle).

Calculating Your Ideal Calorie Range

Your body uses the calories in the food you eat for energy to live (for life-sustaining bodily processes). If you eat more calories than you need for those bodily processes, then you gain weight and those excess calories are stored as fat. (Where you store that fat is genetically determined.)

Today's society is one where tasty and inexpensive high calorie food pervades the environment and makes it incredibly easy to eat excess calories. Combine this with a sedentary lifestyle, and it's no wonder that overweight and obesity are epidemic in the United States. A healthy lifestyle means figuring out how to visually monitor your caloric intake so that it becomes second nature recognizing just "how much is too much."

You can start today to incorporate these tricks to help you manage both sides of the calorie equation.

Curbing your calories in

Foods that are considered high calorie, or calorically dense, have a large number of calories relative to their serving size. Junk food, such as soda and potato chips, typically has a lot of calories with few nutrients. These foods are also known as *empty calorie foods*, which means they have little nutritional value (no vitamins, minerals, antioxidants, or fiber) so you basically get calories without much else.

For example, a 12-ounce can of regular soda provides you with 39 grams of added sugar and 140 liquid calories that you can easily swallow in a few minutes. Many typical American foods have a lot of empty calories. Oils, butter, and other fats; fried foods; and sugary sweets are high-calorie foods. Zero in on your diet where those junk foods may be sneaking in.

TIP

A relatively simple change you can make is to eliminate liquid sugar calories from your diet, such as regular sodas, fruit juices, flavored milks, and other beverages with added sugar. Live by nutritionists' favorite tip: Don't drink your calories.

You can also eat calorically dense food that is very nutritious. For example, peanut butter is a healthy protein choice that also contains a nice amount of good fats and some fiber. Peanut butter is also a good source of magnesium, which is an essential nutrient for people with diabetes. Beware though, two tablespoons pack a huge calorie punch — loaded with as many calories and fat as a candy bar! Discover which of your favorite healthy foods are calorically dense and begin to savor every delicious bite.

One of my goals is to help you eat well and make food choices that promote good health, prevent disease, and assist you in achieving (and maintaining) a healthy weight. This new lifestyle will inevitably result in you looking better, feeling better, and ultimately living better.

Expending your calories out

Weight control is all in the calorie math. To lose weight, you must make changes in both your food intake and exercise patterns such that you reduce your calorie intake below your energy expenditure. When calculating your ideal calorie range to achieve your goals, you need to know a little more about what make ups your energy expenditure side of this equation.

> Weight loss = Weekly calories burned greater than weekly calories eaten

TECHNICAL STUFF

Your body burns calories in several ways. To figure out exactly how many you burn each day, also known as your *total daily energy expenditure (TDEE)*, you need to know your *basal metabolic rate (BMR)* and your general activity level. (The *thermic effect of the food (TEF)* or the calories burned to metabolize the food you eat also contributes to your TDEE, contributing up to 10 percent.)

Your *BMR* is the number of calories your body uses while at rest to do the stuff that keeps you alive like breathing; circulating blood; and controlling body temperature, cell growth, brain and nerve function, and contraction of muscles. Your BMR accounts for roughly 60 percent of your daily calorie expenditure. BMR varies from person to person. Factors affecting BMR include your body weight, your height, your gender, your percent body fat and muscle mass, your body temperature, your age, your hormone levels, and your genetic predisposition. Unfortunately, you don't have much control over your BMR.

Figure 3-1 categorizes the calorie burn side of the equation. The remaining 30 percent of TDEE is physical activity, which then gets broken down into exercise activity thermogenesis (EAT) and nonexercise activity thermogenesis (NEAT). EAT accounts for about 5 percent of TDEE, whereas NEAT can contribute as much as 15 percent. You can see how you have a great deal of control over your dual activity levels, the calorie-burning furnaces: your NEAT and EAT.

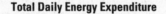

Total Daily Energy Expenditure

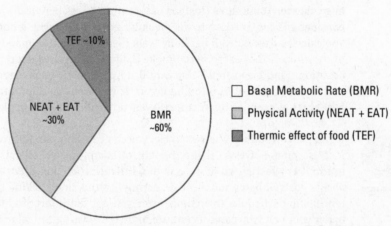

TEF ~10%

NEAT + EAT ~30%

BMR ~60%

☐ Basal Metabolic Rate (BMR)
◩ Physical Activity (NEAT + EAT)
◼ Thermic effect of food (TEF)

FIGURE 3-1: Breaking down your total daily energy expenditure.

© John Wiley & Sons, Inc.

Burning calories through exercise

The burning of calories through physical activity, combined with reducing the number of calories you eat, creates the magical calorie deficit that results in weight loss. You need to consciously make an effort to move more during your days, an action that will make a dent in your NEAT. NEAT is essentially movement you do that isn't formal exercise, such as cleaning the house, shopping for groceries, or even just fidgeting. Take the stairs over the elevator, park farther away from the store, stay away from drive-throughs, and stand more and sit less. All these seemingly small physical efforts add up and can make a huge contribution to your calorie burn. Become a NEAT freak and boost your daily calorie burn!

With planned exercise, or your EAT, your goal should be to find an exercise that you enjoy doing, one that will burn a few hundred daily calories. The number of calories your body burns during exercise depends again on your height, weight, age, body composition, and a bunch of other factors. The calories burned, such as the number that pops up on an exercise machine, is at best a very broad (and very imprecise) estimate.

WEB EXTRAS

If you're curious about how many calories you burn during different types of exercise, you can estimate your calorie expenditure by using a simple online calculator. The Calorie Control Council website has a Get Moving Calculator at `https://caloriecontrol.org/healthy-weight-tool-kit/get-moving-calculator` that allows you to get into the nitty-gritty of what a realistic amount of exercise-and therefore potential calorie burn-is for you and you alone (genius idea):

Consider Kiki's numbers. Kiki weighs 150 pounds. Plug her data into the online calculator and magically see how many calories she burns during her 30-minute dog walk at a moderate pace: 102 calories per walk. If Kiki were to walk her dog every day for 30 minutes (instead of just three times per week) she would make a considerable contribution to her weekly calorie deficit; she'd burn approximately 700 calories a week from her daily walk instead of approximately 300. The moral of the story is that exercise *can* make a difference in the calorie burn side of the equation. Find an exercise that you'll do preferably every day of the week. No marathons required! Flip to Chapter 14 if you want an additional primer on the best types of exercise to accompany your intermittent fasting plan.

REMEMBER

If you plan on adding a new exercise, you can certainly run it through the formula. At this point, however, if the thought of adding a new exercise and practicing intermittent fasting all at once is too difficult, then don't. Focus instead on the doable goals of being more active, eating healthy, and sticking to your intermittent fasting schedule. Over time, after you get the intermittent fasting lifestyle under your belt, you can concentrate more on boosting the calorie burn side of the equation.

Doing the calculations

You can do the calculations and determine just how many daily calories you'll need to take in and burn through exercise in order to create the calorie deficit needed (to lose weight safely). Or, if your goal is to maintain your weight, or even gain muscle mass, you can also calculate what a healthy calorie intake number would be.

WARNING

Your calorie deficit shouldn't be severe. You need to consume enough calories to function well, exercise, and stay healthy. Eating enough calories also helps maintain muscle mass during the weight-loss process.

The first step is to get an estimate of your daily calorie needs for maintaining your current weight. This depends on several factors:

» **Your age:** Enter your age in years.

» **Your height:** Enter your height in feet and inches.

» **Your current weight:** Enter your body weight in pounds.

» **Your gender:** Online calculators require you to input if you are a man or a woman. If you identify your gender as something other than man or woman, for the purposes of online calculations, choose the gender that most matches your body type.

Calculations of how many calories you need per day also require you to input your estimated activity level. Your activity level is generally categorized as follows:

» **Inactive:** Never or rarely include physical activity in your day.

» **Somewhat active:** Include light activity or moderate activity about two to three times a week.

» **Active:** Include at least 30 minutes of moderate activity most days of the week or 20 minutes of vigorous activity at least three days a week.

» **Very active:** Include large amounts of moderate or vigorous activity in your day.

If you fall in the inactive category, I hope this lifestyle plan will help motivate you to move more — not only for the long-term weight loss maintenance benefits but also so you can tap into the significant health benefits an active lifestyle has been proven to provide.

WEB EXTRAS

The easiest way to estimate your calorie range is to use an online calculator. The Mayo Clinic has a simple calorie calculator at `www.mayoclinic.org/` and search for calorie calculator.

TIP

After you have your estimated typical daily calorie needs from your current body weight and activity level, then you can use the Mayo Clinic calculator to see how many more calories you can eat if you increase your activity level. You can also get the big picture of how intermittent fasting reduces your calorie intake and promotes weight loss.

See how this is done using Kiki's goals and activity level. Take Kiki's stats from the previous section, and plug in her age (45), height (5-4), weight (150 pounds), and gender (female). Her activity level is somewhat active (Kiki walks her dog for 30 minutes three times per week).

Her estimated calorie needs are as follows: She needs to eat somewhere around 1850 calories per day (approximately 13,000 calories per week) to maintain her current weight.

REMEMBER

One of the sad facts of life is that when you do lose weight, you need to recalculate the number of calories you can eat to continue your weight-loss journey spiraling downward, because a smaller body has a lower BMR. In other words, the skinnier you get, the less calories you can eat to continue losing weight. The good news is you can offset this by bumping up your activity level.

Consider Kiki again: She wants to lose 10 pounds, and she has chosen to practice the 5:2 intermittent fasting plan (on two nonconsecutive days in a week she confines her eating to one 500 calorie meal; refer to Chapter 12 for more about this plan). Assuming she continues to eat 1,850 calories on five days in a week plus her 1,000 calories (on her two fasting days) gives her a grand total of about 10,250 calories ingested in one week. If she continues with her current activity level, she'll have created a calorie deficit of 2,800 calories per week (presuming she continues her 300 calorie burn per week from her dog walks). Kiki will lose about a pound a week — the recommended safe rate of weight loss.

REMEMBER

Choose an approach to eating (don't call it a diet — it's a lifestyle) that best fits your personality. Part 3 discusses the different fasting plans you may want to consider. Whichever one you choose, ensure that your meals leave you satisfied, not hungry and definitely not deprived.

Following the 80:20 rule

One of the main reason diets fail is because people deprive themselves of the foods they love. When life happens, they go off the diet and gorge on those foods they restricted during the diet. Face it, if you love carbs, there's no way that you'll ever be able to not eat pasta for the next 50 years! The long-term solution and the gold standard of dietary balance and moderation is what nutritionists call the 80:20 rule.

The *80:20 rule*, more formally called the *Pareto principle*, states that, for many events, roughly 80 percent of the effects come from 20 percent of the causes. If you apply this philosophy to your eating regime, you can use it as an approach to healthy eating. The 80:20 rule shows you the way to balance, moderation, and indulging without any feelings of guilt. Don't let perfection be the enemy of the good.

The basic idea of the 80/20 rule as it applies to your intermittent fast is very simple. In order to be healthy and balanced, you don't always have to make 100 percent healthy food choices. Eighty percent will do the trick. You can choose less healthy food and indulge yourself without guilt with the remaining 20 percent. Think of your 20 percent time as the freedom to eat the foods you love that may not be the healthiest. The 80/20 rule is a fantastic way to enjoy your treats and stay on the intermittent fasting train.

TIP

Your indulgences need to be a reasonable portion rather than a free-for-all eat fest. Just because your 20 percent is for treats doesn't mean you can go rogue with the entire pint of ice cream.

Revisit Kiki again: She loves her red wine (she drinks one 8-ounce glass a night) and munches on her nighttime snacks. Kiki has zero intention of giving them up. She is following the 5:2 intermittent fast. On her five non-fasting days, she eats three healthy plant-based meals totaling approximately 1,400 calories. That leaves her with 450 treat calories for nighttime. If she makes her dog walking a daily routine, she gets to add an additional 100 calories to her treats stash or 550 calories per night during her five non-fasting days. Five hundred and fifty calories translate into 8 ounces of red wine (approximately 200 calories) plus an additional 350-calorie high volume, slow-eating snack such as a huge bowl of popcorn. No deprivation here!

WARNING

Red wine in moderation is a heart-healthy habit. However, doctors advise against beginning to drink if you don't already do so. Exercise caution with any alcohol consumption because alcohol carries with it the risk of overindulgence, with many negative health effects. According to the American Heart Association, moderate consumption is one to two drinks per day for men and one drink per day (5 fluid ounces) for women. If you have any doubts about whether it's safe for you to consume wine or any type of alcohol, ask your personal physician.

Trying just one more time

Several intermittent fasting approaches can succeed in helping you attain your goals. Intermittent fasting has many healthful effects on your body such as flipping your metabolic switch and changing your hormonal balance, which contribute to weight loss. But make no mistake about it, intermittent fasting doesn't work through magic, and these plans don't work through some secret bio-hack. Intermittent fasting lifestyles cause weight and body fat loss primarily by creating a sustained calorie deficit.

If you've tried intermittent fasting for a few weeks and haven't lost any weight (or maybe you've even gained a little) despite doing everything by the book, you can easily get discouraged and give up. One of the major mistakes people make when first trying this lifestyle is giving up too soon. This lifestyle takes time to adjust to and for you to see results. If the plan isn't working for you after say six weeks, switch to a different intermittent fasting schedule or better yet, come back to this chapter and do the calorie math. The calculations enable you to pinpoint where the problem areas are in your calorie intake (food consumption) and/or calorie output (exercise). Just remember to keep at it.

Chapter **4**

Understanding the Link Between Weight and Health

I f you're overweight and have been trying to lose weight, you are far from alone. The latest national stats on dieting have found that nearly half of American adults are trying to trim their widening waistlines. This is a smart move — being overweight is harmful to your health.

According to the experts, obesity rates continue to escalate — approximately 72 percent of U.S. adults are now overweight. Add to this statistic the fact that their physical activity rates are abysmally low, and you have the perfect recipe for creating the epidemic of type 2 diabetes that plagues the United States.

REMEMBER

Scientists differentiate between the terms *overweight* and *obese*, using the body mass index (BMI) calculation. *Overweight* is defined as having a BMI between 25 and 29.9. *Obesity* is defined as having a BMI of 30 or more. Both terms are used to identify people who are at risk for health problems from having too much body fat. However, obese generally means a much higher amount of body fat than overweight. Everyone who falls in the obese range is overweight, but not the other way around. Refer to Chapter 2 where I discuss the BMI in greater detail.

Clearly, many Americans need to lose weight. In fact, even a modest weight loss of just 10 percent of your body weight can treat and often reverse the un-healthy conditions associated with being overweight.

Discovering What the Scientists Know about Being Overweight

Everyone needs some body fat for good health. When people eat more calories than they use, their bodies store the extra calories as fat. A couple of pounds of extra body fat is no big deal for most people. The problem arises when people continue this pattern of eating more calories than they burn (creating a *calorie surplus*) over an extended period of time.

More and more fat builds up in the body, and eventually the amount of body fat is so great that it can harm a person's health. Many doctors use the terms *overweight* or *obese* to tell if someone has a greater chance of developing serious weight-related health problems from excess body fat. The good news is, when you lose weight and the closer you can get to a normal weight (a BMI under 25), the greater the health benefits.

REMEMBER

In today's looks-obsessed society, many people are more concerned that being overweight is an appearance issue. But being overweight is a lot more than aesthetics. A BMI higher than 25 is a medical concern because it can seriously affect your health.

If you know that your BMI is above 25 and that the extra poundage is from too much fat and not muscle, then read on to see the toll that this condition can eventually take on your body.

Enumerating the numerous health risks of being overweight

Too much body fat is bad news for both your body and mind. Not only can being overweight make you feel tired and uncomfortable, carrying extra weight also puts added stress on your body, especially the bones and joints of the legs. The more body fat you have, the greater your risk of developing grave health conditions.

TIP

If you're overweight, you may feel perfectly fine. However, the extra body fat puts an insidious strain on your bodily processes. Luckily, it's never too late to make positive lifestyle changes such as following an intermittent fasting plan. This action can prevent additional weight gain and promote loss of body fat, which will prevent or alleviate many of the the following health problems associated with being overweight.

Heart disease

Heart disease is the leading killer of both men and women in the United States. The American Heart Association has now recognized overweight and obesity as a major, independent risk factor for heart disease. Excess body fat taxes the heart. People who have excess body fat — especially if concentrated around the waist — are more likely to have a heart attack than those people at a healthy weight. The good news is, if you're overweight or obese, you can significantly reduce your risk for heart disease by successfully losing weight and keeping it off.

High blood pressure

High blood pressure is also known as the silent killer because it's largely a symptomless disease. The fact that high blood pressure doesn't have symptoms (you can't see or feel it) is what makes high blood pressure so insidious; left untreated, it will kill you. In fact, high blood pressure remains the most common medical diagnosis in the United States and the condition that doctors write the most prescriptions for. It's also the number one cause of stroke and kidney disease and a principal cause of heart disease and blindness.

Overweight people are five times more likely to have high blood pressure than normal weight individuals. The more body fat a person carries, the more blood is needed to provide the tissue with oxygen and nutrients, resulting in higher blood pressure. Researchers have found that extra body fat activates the two underlying origins of elevated pressure: an overactive sympathetic nervous system and an overactive renin (blood pressure hormone) system. The good news is that if you lose body fat, your blood pressure will significantly go down.

Stroke

Every year, more than 800,000 people in the United States have a stroke. Stroke kills almost 130,000 Americans annually and is a leading cause of serious long-term disability. On average, one American dies from stroke every four minutes. If you're overweight, your risk of having a stroke significantly increases because of inflammation occurring in the arteries. Inflammation is partially caused by excess fat and can lead to difficulty in blood flow and an increased risk of blockage in the arteries. Excess body fat has also been shown to increase risk of stroke/transient ischemic attack (also known as a *mini-stroke*).

Insulin resistance and type 2 diabetes

Type 2 diabetes develops when a person has insulin resistance. *Insulin* is the hormone that enables sugar (glucose) to enter cells. *Insulin resistance* means that the body's cells are no longer sensitive to insulin and can't use it correctly. This loss in sensitivity to insulin means the person begins to lose the ability to take in glucose.

Excess body fat, especially around the abdomen, is a major cause of insulin resistance. The development of insulin resistance marks the beginning of diabetes. In time, the resistance to insulin exhausts the pancreas, which may stop producing this hormone entirely, meaning the diabetic must inject insulin. A program of regular exercise and weight loss has been shown to reverse insulin resistance.

Syndrome X

One out of every five individuals who is affected by excess body weight has a metabolic condition known as Syndrome X. *Syndrome X* is a cluster of metabolic factors that increases your risk for disease. The issues that characterize this condition include high blood pressure, insulin resistance, and abdominal belly fat. People with Syndrome X are at a significantly increased risk for developing more serious health problems including heart disease, diabetes, and stroke.

Kidney disease and kidney failure

Being overweight can directly affect your kidneys. Extra body fat forces the kidneys to work harder and filter wastes above the normal level. Over time, this extra work increases the risk for kidney disease. Being overweight is also associated with an increased progression of the disease to kidney failure.

REMEMBER

Losing weight can prevent damage to the kidneys and has also been shown to slow disease progression in people already diagnosed with chronic kidney disease. Trimming down to a healthy body weight can reduce your risk of developing obstructive sleep apnea, increased urine protein excretion, type 2 diabetes, and high blood pressure, which in turn will lower your risk for developing kidney disease.

Cancer

Higher amounts of body fat are associated with increased risks of a number of cancers. Being overweight increases your risk of developing the following types of cancer (Figure 4-1 shows these 13 types of cancers, which account for about 40 percent of all cancer):

- » Meningioma
- » Adenocarcinoma
- » Multiple myeloma
- » Kidney cancer
- » Uterine cancer
- » Ovarian cancer
- » Thyroid cancer

- » Breast cancer
- » Liver cancer
- » Gallbladder cancer
- » Upper stomach cancer
- » Pancreatic cancer
- » Colon and rectal cancer

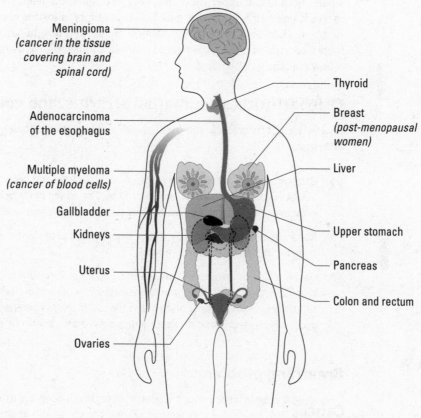

Meningioma
(cancer in the tissue covering brain and spinal cord)

Adenocarcinoma of the esophagus

Multiple myeloma (cancer of blood cells)

Gallbladder

Kidneys

Uterus

Ovaries

Thyroid

Breast (post-menopausal women)

Liver

Upper stomach

Pancreas

Colon and rectum

FIGURE 4-1: Thirteen cancers associated with being overweight.

Source: www.cdc.gov

High cholesterol and blood triglycerides

Abnormal blood fats, also known as *dyslipidemia*, refers to an imbalance of fats circulating in your bloodstream. Being overweight increases the odds of you having a heart attack or stroke by raising the level of artery-clogging blood fats such as triglycerides and LDL cholesterol (which is considered the bad kind of cholesterol). Abdominal obesity also results in reduced levels of HDL cholesterol (the good kind that protects against heart disease).

Gall bladder disease

Gallstones are hardened cholesterol deposits that develop in the gallbladder, a small organ in the upper right abdomen just below the liver. Excess body weight makes it more difficult for the gallbladder to empty, allowing cholesterol-rich bile to accumulate and harden into stones. Being overweight also exposes you to increased risk of gallstone-related complications and *cholecystectomy* (surgical removal of the gall bladder).

Osteoarthritis, rheumatoid arthritis, and gout

Excess weight increases the risk of developing the following three types of arthritis:

>> *Osteoarthritis* occurs when the cartilage that cushions and protects the ends of bones in your joints wears down over time. The added body weight puts more pressure and stress on weight-bearing joints such as knees and hips.

>> *Rheumatoid arthritis,* an autoimmune disorder, is caused when the body fat releases inflammatory compounds.

>> *Gout* is a kind of arthritis characterized by an excess amount of uric acid in the blood. Symptoms often include intense episodes of painful swelling and tenderness in joints, most often in the big toe. If you're overweight, your body produces more uric acid and your kidneys have a tougher time eliminating it.

Breathing problems

Overweight people have a much higher risk of developing asthma, especially people with a BMI over 30. Extra weight around the chest and abdomen constrict the lungs and make it more difficult to breathe. Fat tissue produces inflammatory substances that cause the inner lining of the airways to swell and mucus to be produced, which makes the airways more sensitive to asthma triggers.

Sleep problems

Being overweight increases the likelihood of suffering from sleep-disordered breathing, known as *sleep apnea.* In turn, people with sleep apnea have a greater risk of high blood pressure, irregular heart rhythms, and stroke. Sleeping less also gives you more time for late night snacking, contributing to weight gain.

Nonalcoholic fatty liver disease

Excess body fat, especially in the abdominal area, increases the likelihood of developing what is termed *nonalcoholic fatty liver disease (NAFLD).* NAFLD begins with the abnormal accumulation of deposits of fat in the liver cells. Liver cells normally help to process and regulate the amount of sugar and fat in the blood. However, extra body fat overwhelms the cells triggering the formation of fatty deposits. In fact, the BMI correlates with the amount of liver damage, that is, the greater the BMI the greater the damage.

Polycystic ovarian syndrome

Polycystic ovarian syndrome (PCOS) is a hormonal reproductive disorder, extremely common in overweight women, especially women with insulin resistance. PCOS refers to the appearance of small cysts along the outer edge of the enlarged ovaries of women with this condition. Excess insulin circulating in the blood results in overproduction of *androgens* (male sex hormones). Too much of this type of hormone prevents ovulation.

Psychological effects

Being overweight predisposes you to suffering psychological ills. A poor self-image, physical inactivity, the biological disruptions caused by excess body fat, and the social stigma related to being overweight all contribute to a predisposition to mental illness.

Reduced length and quality of life

Overweight and obesity are serious health concerns. The poor mental health, the reduced quality of life from many of the diseases and disorders that I mention in the previous sections, and the predisposition to develop the leading causes of death in the United States and worldwide clearly reduce length and quality of life.

IDENTIFYING THE CAUSES OF CALORIE SURPLUS

People become overweight from creating an extended calorie surplus. If you've gained weight, it may be because you're making unhealthy food choices (like fast food) and poor behavioral habits (such as eating mindlessly in front of the TV or while driving in your car). High-calorie, low-nutrient snacks and beverages, huge portions of food, and less-active lifestyles all contribute to the obesity epidemic.

You may be someone who turns to food for emotional reasons, such as when you feel upset, anxious, sad, stressed out, or even bored. If so, try writing the answers to these questions in your journal, an exercise in self-examination that can help you identify and overcome this obstacle to achieving your healthy lifestyle goals:

- Do you tend to overeat in response to emotions? If yes, what emotions are your trigger?
- What seems to be the root cause?
- What and where do you eat?

I also suggest you flip to Chapter 2, where I give you more journaling exercises to work on as you progress through your intermittent fasting lifestyle.

Consider the following, which are things that may lead to your calorie surplus:

- Eating a poor diet and making unhealthy food choices
- Eating out often and chowing down on oversized restaurant food portions
- Inheriting being overweight or obese
- Feeling negative emotions like stress, boredom, sadness, or anger, that may influence eating habits
- Living an inactive lifestyle:
  - Spending too time in front of a screen — watching television, playing video games, working on a computer
  - Choosing to be more sedentary (driving rather than walking, taking the elevator instead of the stairs, and so on)
  - Not exercising enough

Seeing why where you store your fat matters

There is a problem with relying on traditional BMI measurements to determine whether someone is overweight or obese. These measurements ignore many people who have excessive body fat that puts them at risk of various health conditions. There is a new term being used in the medical world, namely, *overfat*. Overfat describes an overload of fat that builds up in certain parts of the body (the midsection), and it can affect even individuals who are of normal weight or BMI. Such a buildup of fat can pose serious metabolic threats to one's health such as insulin resistance, high blood pressure, heart disease, stroke, and even cancer. In this section, I explore the dangers of the so-called overfat pandemic that is currently sweeping the United States and the myriad health risks of excess body belly fat and what it really means to be overfat.

REMEMBER

Concerning body fat, location counts. Your body shape can say a lot about your health and your hormones. In other words, fat isn't created equal. If you know you're overweight, focus on where you're carrying that excess body fat, which will give you a better idea of what type of fat you have. The two types of fat are as follows:

>> **Subcutaneous:** The jiggly fat located just under the skin you can pinch with your fingers and the type aesthetically bothersome

>> **Visceral:** Fat lying deep within the abdomen, surrounding the organs

Women, when they're younger, tend to store subcutaneous fat around the hips and thighs, giving them a pear-shaped physique, mostly due to the impact of estrogen on fat distribution. A pear-shaped fat distribution is healthier; however, this fat is obstinate and is typically the hardest type of fat to lose. Pear-shaped women are better protected from metabolic diseases like diabetes compared to big-bellied people. Stubborn subcutaneous fat is not as dangerous for your health as the visceral fat that lives deep down within the abdominal cavity.

When women go through menopause, the location of where the body tends to store fat shifts, so that more body fat ends up around the middle and in the waist and tummy area. The pattern of storing fat around the middle (an apple shape) is much more strongly linked to chronic health problems than storing excess fat in the hips and thighs (a pear-shaped physique). Fat that builds up around your middle and deep within your abdomen places you at higher risk of heart disease, syndrome X, and type 2 diabetes. I discuss apple and pear shapes in Chapter 2 in greater detail.

When men gain weight, they tend to store more fat deep in the midsection of the body, which is where the dangerous type of fat lives (refer to Figure 4-2). Visceral fat penetrates way down inside, enveloping the visceral organs such as the liver, heart, kidneys, pancreas, and intestines. Visceral fat is also known as a *deep fat* or *intra-abdominal fat.* Check out the nearby sidebar for more about visceral fat.

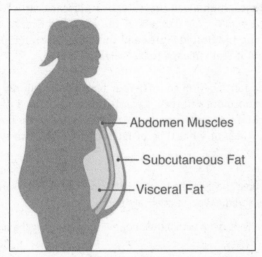

Abdomen Muscles

Subcutaneous Fat

Visceral Fat

FIGURE 4-2:
Visceral fat versus subcutaneous fat.

Source: Used with permission from © logo3in1

REMEMBER

Women tend to have more subcutaneous fat relative to men who carry a higher percentage of more dangerous visceral fat. That is until menopause, when a woman's visceral fat storage increases as do their health risks. How do you know if you have a dangerous level of visceral fat? Your best clue is your waist size. Instead of trying to figure out how much of your visible belly fat is visceral and how much is subcutaneous, just realize that any large waistline poses a risk and is unhealthy. Waist size rises as visceral fat deposits increase. For women, a waist circumference over 35 inches is a red flag, while men should be concerned as waist size rises above 40 inches.

VISCERAL FAT'S UGLY SIDE

Visceral fat is insidious and causes disease because it releases inflammatory chemicals that fuel inflammation. Scientists know that inflammation is the driver of most diseases. The good news is visceral fat is easier to lose than subcutaneous fat through lifestyle changes, such as following an intermittent fasting plan and exercising.

Here are the specific health hazards of high levels of visceral fat:

- **Diabetes:** Visceral fat plays a large role in causing insulin resistance, which means a heightened risk for developing type 2 diabetes.

- **Inflammation:** Visceral fat produces hormonal and inflammatory molecules that get dumped directly into the liver, leading to dangerous inflammation and hormone-disrupting reactions.

- **Increased appetite:** Visceral fat increases the brain's hormonal messengers, the ones prompting people to eat more.

- **Increased risk of heart disease and stroke:** Visceral fat play havoc with your blood markers of cardiovascular disease such as increasing triglycerides, increasing blood pressure, and raising cholesterol.

- **Increased risk of dementia:** Visceral fat promotes a greater risk of developing dementia than those people with smaller bellies.

- **Depression:** Visceral fat changes the level of brain neurotransmitters, which can negatively impact mood and increase risk of depression.

Beating the Odds of Inheriting the Fat Genes

Genes also play a role in becoming overweight. They affect how much fat a person stores and where it's stored. Overweight tends to run in families; some people have a genetic tendency to gain weight more easily than others. Genes strongly influence body type and size, meaning if your mother has an apple shape and is overweight, you may have inherited her shape.

Two people living in the same environment (tons of high calorie food and living a sedentary life) may react differently. Both will most likely become overweight, but they won't have the same body fat distribution or suffer the same health problems. This variation in how people respond to the same environment is explained by the role genes play in how a person becomes overweight.

If you have inherited any of these so-called *fat genes*, does that mean all is lost and you're predisposed to becoming and remaining overweight? No! Many people who carry these genes don't become overweight, and healthy lifestyles can easily counteract the potential genetic effects. Your genetic makeup may make it slightly more difficult to lose weight by giving you an increased appetite and reduced metabolic rate, however, following a consistent healthy intermittent fasting plan combined with daily physical activity can defeat your genetic predisposition.

REMEMBER

Your heredity is *not* your destiny! Creating a healthy environment and lifestyle can counteract gene-related risks. The contribution of genes to risk of becoming overweight is small, while the contribution of your toxic food and activity environment is huge.

Getting going on your intermittent fasting lifestyle of choice will immediately begin to change your body. When you start to lose the fat and even gain some muscle, your wellness will dramatically improve.

2
Grasping the Health Benefits of Intermittent Fasting

Discover how much science there is backing up the safety and efficacy of following an intermittent fasting plan for better health.

Observe how flipping your metabolic switch is the mechanism linked to so many positive changes in your body.

See how scientists paint a crystal-clear picture of why this lifestyle works to help you achieve your weight, health, and anti-aging goals.

Examine the multitude of health benefits gained specifically from the practice of intermittent fasting.

Determine if intermittent fasting is right for you.

Identify who should *never* practice intermittent fasting.

Chapter **5**

Navigating the Science of Intermittent Fasting

The practice of intermittent fasting is easier to stick to than traditional diet plans. But that alone doesn't account for its staying power. Intermittent fasting also has its share of clinical studies to back it up.

In this chapter, I explain exactly how intermittent fasting impacts your body. You can discover firsthand how the science does indeed support all the hype. Although intermittent fasting may seem simple in theory — cycle through periods of fasting and periods of eating normally — how it affects the body, your metabolism, and even your quality of sleep is a bit more complicated. The inner workings of what goes on in the body during fasting is nothing short of fascinating.

THE EVOLUTION OF INTERMITTENT FASTING

Intermittent fasting isn't the first dietary pattern of eating to excite researchers. Scientists actually have studied fasting for 100 years.

Before intermittent fasting, Scientists studied *calorie restriction* and used the term CR to define the reduction of calorie intake over an extended amount of time. In the CR studies, they found lab animals, usually mice, whose daily calorie intake was restricted by 20 to 40 percent, lived longer and had a lower chance of chronic illness and disease than their free-eating counterparts. The revelation was extraordinary! Eating less than the body apparently needs is a healthy strategy. CR was used to study the biology of aging, as it has remarkable effects on aging and life span, at least in mice. The question was, would CR work in humans?

In 2002, researchers conducted a CR study on humans (143 normal and slightly overweight men and women between the ages of 21 and 51). They ate 25 percent fewer calories than usual for two years. The conclusion was striking: During the study period, the people following CR had aged more slowly than those in the control group. Furthermore, blood pressure, cholesterol, glucose, insulin, and other disease biomarkers fell, possibly lowering their risk for heart disease, cancer and diabetes.

Fast forward to studies in humans specifically involving intermittent fasting protocols, as opposed to CR, and you'll understand the changes that are happening in your body during your intermittent fasting journey. See exactly what goes on in the human body during the fasted state. These changes all contribute to the disease protection and longevity that intermittent fasting will provide you.

Discerning What The Scientists Know about Intermittent Fasting

The study of the effects of different intermittent fasting protocols on the human body is still in its infancy. Although much of the research has been in animals, promising well-designed human trials are emerging. In fact, a growing body of research specifically is investigating some of the more popular versions of intermittent fasting that is shedding light on the inner workings of intermittent fasting in humans. Intermittent fasting is a hot topic in the research world. Here I get you up to speed on what the scientists presently know.

How intermittent fasting affects your cells and hormones

The shear act of restricting food and calories for an extended period of time sets off a host of bodily processes on the cellular and molecular level. During the fasting state, the following actions occur.

Cells

Genes are activated that direct cells to preserve resources. Rather than grow and divide, cells in the fasting mode are stalled. In this state, they're mostly resistant to disease and stress. The changes in the function of these genes promote longevity.

Cells enter into autophagy, a kind of cellular housekeeping sparking cellular rejuvenation. *Autophagy* is that self-cleaning cellular process that boosts brain functioning and maybe even longevity. When cells are in fasting mode and don't have to work to break down food, they pause their usual tasks and stop dividing. Instead, they work on repairing and recycling damaged components and digest dead or toxic cell matter. Chapter 6 provides more info about autophagy.

Cells activate pathways that enhance their defenses against oxidative and metabolic stress. *Oxidative stress* is one of the major contributing factors for aging and the development of many chronic diseases. Oxidative stress involves unstable molecules called *free radicals,* which react with other important molecules (like protein and DNA) and injure them. Fighting off free radicals also leads to reduced inflammation — a major cause of many diseases.

Your entire body minimizes the building processes (such as making new cells), instead, favoring cellular repair systems. This transition is what improves health and disease resistance. After you begin to eat again, your cells have adapted to make better use of the fat, carbs, and proteins you ingest.

Hormones

Intermittent fasting decreases some hormones and increases others. Intermittent fasting *decreases* the production of the following:

>> **Insulin:** Intermittent fasting keeps insulin levels low for most of the day, because insulin is released when you eat. Many prediabetics have a condition known as *insulin resistance,* meaning their insulin isn't effective in facilitating blood sugar entering the cells. Intermittent fasting improves the actions of insulin, making cells more sensitive to the hormone. An increase in insulin sensitivity causes insulin and blood sugar levels to drop dramatically. Lower insulin levels make stored body fat more accessible. Lower insulin levels help drive weight loss.

>> **IGF-1:** This hormone is key to cellular growth. IGF-1 increases cancer risk and accelerates aging when not suppressed. High levels of IGF-1, which is a protein produced by the liver, specifically raise the risks of colorectal, breast, and prostate cancer. Low levels of IGF-1 reduce those risks.

Meanwhile, here are a couple hormones that intermittent fasting *boosts*:

>> **Glucagon:** *Glucagon* is a hormone produced by the pancreas with opposite effects to its pancreatic twin, insulin. Glucagon raises metabolic rate, decreases appetite, and increases the breakdown of body fat for use as energy.

>> **Human growth hormone (HGH):** HGH, produced by your pituitary gland, plays a key role in growth, body composition, cell repair, and metabolism, boosting muscle growth, strength, and exercise performance, while helping you recover from injury and disease. Insulin spikes (with regular eating patterns) can disrupt your natural human growth hormone production.

>> **Norepinephrine:** Also called *noradrenaline,* your adrenal glands and nerves release this hormone that functions both as a hormone and *neurotransmitter* (a substance that sends signals between nerve cells). The general role of norepinephrine is to mobilize the brain and body for action. Intermittent fasting not only boosts the production but also the release of this fat-burning hormone. Norepinephrine is the main driver of the increased metabolic rate observed with intermittent fasting.

REMEMBER

As I discuss in Chapter 3, weight loss occurs when you create a calorie deficit. The alteration in hormones will increase your metabolic rate. In other words, intermittent fasting works on both sides of the calorie equation. It boosts your metabolic rate (increases calories out) and reduces the amount of food you eat (reduces calories in) — a double weight-loss whammy! Reduced insulin levels, higher HGH levels, and an increased amount of circulating norepinephrine all increase the breakdown of body fat and facilitate its use for energy.

Flipping your metabolic switch

Metabolic switching is the term used to describe the point during fasting when cells have used up their stores of rapidly accessible, sugar-based fuel, and begin converting fat into energy in a slower metabolic process. Metabolic switching triggers the age-old adaptation to periods of food scarcity during the days of the hunter-gatherers. No food for days on end meant the body had to adapt to utilizing fat stores for energy in lieu of carbohydrates. Furthermore, the fasted state led to improved brain function, enabling humans to devise creative ways to overcome the physical and mental challenges of stalking prey.

The beauty of intermittent fasting is its ability to prompt your body to metabolically switch it up, meaning burn up fat stores for energy. This is a time-limited period of ketosis, meaning when your body goes from using glucose (blood sugar) as a fuel source to tapping into fat stores and creating ketones from the fat (a chemical derived from fat) for energy. You may recognize the word ketones from the popular Keto Diet. (Read more about this diet in Chapter 17.)

REMEMBER

During a period of fasting, the decreasing insulin levels cause cells to release their glucose stores as energy. After about ten hours of no food, your stores of glucose are depleted. With its tanks of glucose empty, the body resorts to dipping into the endless amount of stored fat (in fat cells) as an energy source. Fat cells break down the fat and release it into the bloodstream where it travels to the liver to be converted into more usable energy in the form of ketones. Ketones then circulate throughout the body and are the major source of energy for your cells during the fasted state.

TIP

To ensure that you're flipping your metabolic switch during your intermittent fast, do not eat or drink any calorie containing food during your fasting windows.

Understanding Why Intermittent Fasting Works

Fasting in the historical sense means starving oneself for long periods of time. Long-term fasts are dangerous and elicit different effects on the body compared to intermittent fasting protocols. Within the first ten hours or so of calorie deprivation, the body depletes its blood sugar stored in the muscles and the liver (drains the sugar tanks) and switches to the use of ketones and fat for energy (the metabolic switch).

After a few days of fasting, the body begins to break down protein within muscles and fat to produce energy. Meanwhile, hormonal reactions will fluctuate. It's well established that very long periods without food can cause a sizable drop in metabolism. This *starvation mode* is a set of adaptive biochemical and physiological changes that reduce metabolism in response to starvation, a phenomenon you definitely want to avoid. Short-term fasting does not put your body into starvation mode. Instead, your metabolism increases significantly.

WARNING

Intermittent fasting involves only short-term periods of fasting — the amount proven to elicit health-promoting physiological responses. None of the intermittent fasts in this book promote fasting for longer than 36 hours. If you fast much longer, the metabolism boosting effects can reverse. What's more, long term fasts that trigger the starvation mode *aren't* safe.

Fasting intermittently coaxes the body to make changes and operate more efficiently. The different phases your body enters during your fasts is the catalyst for creating the phenomenal health benefits associated with this lifestyle. The process behind the magic is intriguing. Here I take a closer look at what goes on in your body when you begin to fast.

Illuminating the three metabolic states

To fully comprehend intermittent fasting, you need to understand the three metabolic states, which the following sections discuss in greater detail. The following sections discuss these three metabolic states. During any given day, your metabolism typically switches between the fed state and postabsorptive (after food has been digested) states.

The fed state

Also called the *absorptive state*, the *fed state* happens right after you eat — when your body is digesting the food and absorbing its nutrients. As soon as you see or smell food, your mouth may start to water, and digestion has already begun. When the body is fed, glucose (the blood sugar from carbohydrates), fats, and proteins are absorbed across the intestinal membrane and enter the bloodstream to be used immediately for fuel or in the case of protein, used for muscle growth and repair.

If you exert energy shortly after eating, your body will process and immediately use the dietary fats and sugars that were just ingested for energy. If not needed, the excess glucose is stored in the liver and muscle cells, or as fat in fat (adipose) tissue. Release of digested nutrients into the bloodstream stimulates the pancreas to release the hormone insulin. Insulin stimulates the uptake of blood sugar by liver cells, muscle cells, and fat cells.

The postabsorptive state

The *postabsorptive state* happens when the food has been digested, absorbed, and stored. No more nutrients are entering the bloodstream from the digestive system. Sugar concentration in the blood drops and the pancreas stops releasing insulin and starts releasing a different hormone, called glucagon. *Glucagon* directs the liver and muscle cells to release stored blood sugar back into the bloodstream for energy. The postabsorptive state is therefore the metabolic state occurring after digestion when food is no longer the body's source of energy, and it must rely on stored blood sugar for energy.

The fasted state

This state occurs when the body has depleted all its glucose stores. Shifting into the fat-burning state known as ketosis occurs, after your body burns through your glycogen stores (the tanks of sugar stored in your muscles and liver). This is when the metabolic switch occurs. Refer to the section, "Flipping your metabolic switch," earlier in this chapter.

The first priority for survival is to provide enough blood sugar or fuel for the brain (the brain must be supplied with fuel in the form of glucose or ketones, although sugar is the preferred food for the brain). The second priority is the conservation of amino acids for proteins. Therefore, the body uses ketones to satisfy the energy needs of the brain and other blood sugar–dependent organs and to maintain proteins in the cells. In the event that you fast too long, the body goes into starvation mode and begins to break down vital organs and muscle tissue as a fuel source.

It's important to understand that these highly orchestrated physiological events triggered during the fasted state carry over into the fed state to heighten mental and physical performance as well as disease resistance.

Examining the important role of ketones

For the brief period of time your body is in the fasted state, many physiological processes are at work that have healing properties. In addition to autophagy, another process going on is the metabolizing of fat in the liver that releases chemicals called ketones. *Ketones* circulate throughout the body and have many positive actions apart from serving as an alternative fuel source.

Ketones regulate the expression and activity of many proteins and molecules that are known to influence health and aging. Ketones specifically dampen inflammation, the condition associated with promotion of chronic disease. Ketones also interact with muscle cells to improve insulin sensitivity, reducing blood sugar levels.

Ketones are probably most recognized for their healthful effect on brain function. Ketones have a neuroprotective effect, shielding the brain against age-related cognitive decline. It has been known for 50 years that ketones can benefit people with epilepsy and reduce seizure frequency. Ketones, most notably a ketone called *beta-hydroxybutyrate*, has been shown to increase production of brain-derived neurotrophic factor (BDNF), the protein that keeps your brain strong and resistant to neurodegenerative disorders (Alzheimer's disease and Parkinson's disease are the two most common neurodegenerative disorders).

REMEMBER

Switching back and forth between fasting and healthful feeding is the key to providing the unique benefits of intermittent fasting. Prolonged ketosis, such as occurs when you follow a Keto Diet, is a flawed approach to long-term health because the diet itself has been linked to digestive and gall bladder disorders as well as a reduced ability to exercise. People who follow a high-fat, low-carb fad diet for prolonged periods have been shown to be at increased risk for cardiovascular disease and premature death.

Discovering the facts on fat

Like it or not, your fat cells are with you for life — even if you lose weight. When you lose weight, your fats cells (also known as *adipocytes*) simply shrink in size. Fat cells are very flexible, able to grow or shrink dramatically, and can change in size by up to a factor of 50! Most fat cells are created during childhood, stabilizing in early adulthood. Unfortunately, new research shows that although you can't get rid of the cells themselves, (unless you resort to liposuction), if you continue to overeat, the number of fat cells in your lower body is capable of increasing throughout life. In adults, fat-cell number increases in lower body depots after only eight weeks of increased food intake.

When you fast, you increase the amount of fat in the fat cells burned for energy. Over the long term, and if you've succeeded in creating a sustained calorie deficit (you routinely burned more calories than you consumed), you'll reduce the size of your fat cells. Chapter 4 explains the two types of fat in greater detail.

TIP

Just make sure that you don't refill your fat cells by reverting back to old habits. Permanent weight loss requires making healthy changes to your lifestyle and food choices. Here are tips for keeping the weight off:

>> **Practice daily exercise:** Flip to Chapter 14 for more information on the benefits of adding exercise to your intermittent fasting plan.

>> **Slow and steady wins the race:** Refer to Chapter 2 to see what a healthy weight range is for you.

>> **Continue to set goals to keep you motivated**: I discuss setting goals in Chapter 2.

>> **Find a cheering section:** Chapter 24 gives you some tips on finding and using support. Use your toolbox in Chapter 23 to keep you on track.

>> **Get plenty of good quality sleep.** I discuss the importance of getting a good night's sleep in the "Circling the Circadian Rhythm Connection" section later in this chapter.

REMEMBER

Intermittent fasting is here to stay because it's flexible. You can choose an intermittent fasting practice and nutrient plan that fits your lifestyle. You may first choose a plan to help you lose the flab, but soon, I guarantee, you'll make it a routine way of life as you tap into the notable physiological effects such as gaining more energy, inner calm, and mental clarity.

Revving up your metabolic rate

Your *metabolism* is the sum total of all the complex biological processes your body performs to turn the calories you eat and drink into energy. People with a higher metabolic rate can eat more calories to sustain their body weight than people with a lower metabolic rate.

Intermittent fasting affects your *metabolic rate,* depending on the length of the fast. So how does intermittent fasting affect metabolism? Intermittent fasts are short-term fasts. Contrary to what many believe, short-term fasts have been proven to boost metabolism by 3.6 to as much as 14 percent! This phenomenon is primarily due to the drastic increase in blood levels of norepinephrine, released during fasting periods. Refer to the section, "How intermittent fasting affects your cells and hormones," earlier in this chapter for more about this hormone.

Circling the Circadian Rhythm Connection

The *circadian rhythm* — also known as your *body clock* — is a 24-hour biological cycle that occurs in every cell of the body. The circadian rhythm drives your physiology, from when you sleep, to your hormone levels, to when you should eat. The sun is what sets your circadian rhythm. That rhythm expects you to eat during the day when the sun is shining and fast in the darkness — the way caveman ancestors did before there was artificial light. Your body clock is synchronized with the surrounding environment by exposure to the sun and the timing of meals.

A study published in the journal *Cell Metabolism* compared pre-diabetic men practicing intermittent fasting with an eating window from 8 a.m. to 3 p.m. with pre-diabetic men eating a regular American diet from 8 a.m. to 8 p.m. (both diets were calculated to maintain body weight) for five weeks. Only the early intermittent fasting group showed remarkable health improvements: improved blood pressure, decreased oxidative stress and increased insulin sensitivity. According to the researchers, nighttime is for resting, not eating.

Another study published in *the Journal of Human Nutrition and Diet* analyzed the role of eating all your calories during daylight hours versus eating most of them during evening hours. The evidence showed that people who eat most of their calories during daylight hours tend to be leaner than people who eat most of their calories in the evening (these people had a much higher risk of overweight and obesity). The conclusion was that circadian rhythms play a critical role in the physiological processes involved in energy metabolism and energy balance. It's healthier to eat during daylight hours — in sync with natural circadian rhythm.

REMEMBER

The key is consistency. Another superb health benefit to intermittent fasting is it resets your body clock and your sleep cycle, thereby improving quality of sleep. A good night's sleep is just as important as regular exercise and a nutritious diet in keeping you healthy. According to the National Sleep Foundation, a healthy night's sleep means you fall asleep within a half an hour of putting your head on the pillow and stay asleep with no more than one awakening (that you quickly fall back asleep from). Here are a few of the health gains from getting a good night's sleep:

>> **Stress reducer:** Lack of sleep increases the body's production of stress hormones, which are a natural result of today's fast-paced lifestyles. Deep and regular sleep can help mitigate this stress hormone production. Lack of sleep can make you more agitated. The better you sleep, the better your ability to stay calm, controlled, and happy.

>> **Better cardiovascular health:** High blood pressure significantly increases your risk of heart attacks and stroke. Getting plenty of restful sleep encourages a constant state of relaxation that can help reduce blood pressure and generally keep it under control. A regular sleep pattern can help to lower the levels of stress and inflammation to your cardiovascular system, which in turn can reduce your chances of heart disease.

>> **Help with weight control and prevention of diabetes:** Studies have shown that poor sleep habits contribute to weight gain. A good night's sleep can help you keep your weight under control by regulating the hormones that affect your appetite and reducing your cravings for high calorie foods. Some research studies have shown that not getting enough sleep may lead to type 2 diabetes by affecting how your body processes glucose.

TIP

Here are a few ways to help you get a better night's sleep:

>> **Change your environment:** Make your sleeping area dark, quiet, very comfortable and temperature controlled. Calm yourself before sleep by taking a hot bath, reading, meditating or taking any other action that relaxes you.

>> **Prepare early for your night's sleep:** Try to keep your sleep and wake times a consistent ritual. Don't nap during the day and refrain from caffeine, eating and alcohol before bed.

>> **Manipulate your light sources:** Increase your light (sun and artificial) exposure during daylight hours and avoid blue light (the kind of light electronic devices like smartphones and computers emit) exposure in the evening.

Chapter **6**

Identifying the Health Benefits to Intermittent Fasting

No doubt about it, scientists are on board with intermittent fasting as more and more scientific data accumulates proving that adhering to this lifestyle results in a multitude of impressive health benefits. In fact, research shows intermittent fasting is a highly effective weight-loss strategy. However, you should know that intermittent fasting's benefits go far beyond weight loss. You can even garner a wealth of health dividends derived from intermittent fasting by following the plan and simply maintaining your normal body weight.

Intermittent fasting has become a popular lifestyle trend in the health and fitness world, where healthy, fit, and lean people adhere to the program to tap into the remarkable health benefits this lifestyle confers. Although false rumors abound — that intermittent fasting is harmful — on the contrary, short-term (intermittent) fasting has powerful benefits for your body and mind such as lowering inflammation, slowing aging, and giving you a stronger brain.

This chapter reviews how and why intermittent fasting is Mother Nature's best prescription for a longer, healthier life and takes you on a tour of the extraordinary health gains that practicing intermittent fasting affords you. Intermittent fasting is the body's built-in fixer.

Here I discuss how intermittent fasting can prevent or reverse diabetes, weight gain, DNA damage, and other artifacts of aging. I explain the science of how a regular practice can delay or prevent the onset of age-related diseases, such as cancer and neurodegenerative diseases, like Alzheimer's. I also examine how intermittent fasting shapes brain health by enhancing learning and memory. Live longer, live better, and increase your life span with intermittent fasting by fighting aging, cancer, cardiovascular diseases, and neurodegenerative diseases.

Comprehending Why Intermittent Fasting Is a Powerful Weight-Loss Tool

Weight loss is the most common reason for people to try intermittent fasting, but is it effective? The numbers are in. Numerous studies show intermittent fasting is a very powerful weight-loss tool. The main reason is that it helps you eat fewer calories by skipping meals during the fasting periods. By crafting a schedule where you eat fewer meals, intermittent fasting will lead to an automatic reduction in calorie intake. Restricting your meals and snacks to whatever intermittent plan you choose will naturally diminish your calorie intake, promoting a perpetual calorie deficit, which is the key to weight loss.

Intermittent fasting promotes fat loss beyond the food intake side of the calorie equation. These other metabolic factors are what make intermittent fasting so magical not only as a weight loss tool but also for what goes on in the body during the fasting state.

Creating a sustainable calorie deficit

If you want to lose weight, you need to create a sustainable calorie deficit, meaning you take in fewer calories than your body expends over the long run. Unlike conventional calorie restriction diets, intermittent fasting focuses mainly on *when* you eat and not so much *what* you eat. The tremendous appeal of using intermittent fasting as a weight-loss program is the lack of a huge focus on calorie counting and none of the deprivation (banning favorite foods forever) associated with traditional diets.

A major reason intermittent fasting promotes fat loss is the intricate mechanisms your body resorts to during the fasted state. Intermittent fasting increases levels of *norepinephrine,* a hormone and neurotransmitter that boosts your metabolism resulting in an increased calorie burn. Human growth hormone surges, contributing even further to a bump in your metabolic rate. Human growth hormone is an amazing hormone that also encourages burning of fat, preserving of lean muscle mass, enhancing cellular repair, and helping to slow the aging process. Furthermore, this eating pattern results in reduced levels of *insulin,* the pancreatic hormone involved in blood sugar management and fat deposition. Decreased insulin levels accelerate fat burning to promote weight loss. By helping you eat fewer and burn more calories, intermittent fasting causes weight loss by changing both sides of the calorie equation.

WARNING

The primary reason for intermittent fasting's weight loss success is that the plans help you eat fewer calories overall. (Part 3 discusses the different intermittent fasting plans.) If you binge and eat massive amounts during your eating periods, you probably won't lose any weight at all and may even gain some.

A scientific review published in the journal *Translational Research,* compared intermittent fasting with traditional diets. Regular calorie-restricted diets (spanning over 3 to 12 weeks) were contrasted with programs of intermittent fasting lasting the same time periods. The intermittent fasting plans showed similar weight loss (up to 8 percent) and decreases in body fat by (up to 16 percent) compared to the traditional diets. However, the intermittent fasting was much more effective in helping people retain their lean body mass (muscle) compared to regular dieters. Muscle is the human body's metabolic furnace. Lose muscle mass and your metabolic rate drops. This translates into a vicious cycle of weight regain because now you must eat fewer calories to maintain your weight. If you keep eating the same amount and you have less muscle mass to burn those calories, you end up gaining weight over time.

Losing the fat and gaining muscle

Maintaining lean body mass and losing body fat during a weight-loss program should be the ultimate goal. Intermittent fasting maintains muscle mass compared to other reduced calorie diets. This reason harks back to the short-term fasting practiced by your Paleolithic hunter-gatherer ancestors. Maintenance of muscle mass (and fitness) during short periods of fasting allowed humans to survive spells of food shortages.

Weight loss and weight-loss maintenance plans should reduce body fat stores and, as much as possible, preserve muscle mass. This strategy maintains physical function and lessens or even prevents the associated decline in metabolic rate, which help to prevent rebound weight gain. The ideal weight-loss program promotes a safe rate of weight loss of 1 to 2 pounds per week — almost entirely composed of body fat — a side effect of intermittent fasting that drastically increases its appeal.

KETONES — AN ENERGY SOURCE DURING FASTING

When you aren't eating, your body must draw on its internal energy stores. The body favors the use of sugar as its primary fuel source — especially if plenty of carbs and protein are provided in your diet. In fact, some cells in your body, such as brain cells, prefer energy only from glucose. However, during fasting periods, when the sugar supply has been drained, fat is converted by the liver into ketone bodies. *Ketones* serve as a major source of energy for many tissues, especially the brain, during fasting. This energy source transition is referred to as *flipping your metabolic switch,* which I discuss in greater detail in Chapter 5.

In effect, fat in the form of ketones serves as an alternative energy source to maintain normal brain cell metabolism during fasting periods. Without having that alternative source, your brain would be extremely vulnerable, especially if you didn't consume enough calories. In that situation, your own muscle mass would be broken down rapidly and converted into glucose to feed your sugar-hungry brain. The ability of your brain to use a backup source of energy in times of famine is an extraordinary evolutionary phenomenon derived from humankind's Paleolithic hunter-gatherer ancestors need to survive spells of food shortages. Ketones allowed humans to keep up their strength and mental acuity and to survive. The ketone alternative energy system, in effect, prevented the human race from becoming extinct.

Flipping your metabolic switch during intermittent fasting is quite different from following a ketogenic diet. *Keto Diets* are very low-carb, high-protein diets that push the body into an extended period (weeks to months) of ketosis — an *unhealthy* state. The intermittent fasting plans in this book suggest that during your eating periods you follow a *healthy* plant-based, whole foods Mediterranean diet, triggering use of ketones only during limited time periods — only during your fasting windows.

TIP

The best way to concurrently lose fat and gain muscle is to follow a healthy eating intermittent fasting plan with a small calorie deficit and combine this program with a strength training exercise regime geared toward increasing muscle. Flip to Chapter 14 where you can read about choosing an exercise program that's best for you to add to your intermittent fasting plan and achieve your personal goals.

Seeing how intermittent fasting targets belly fat

Belly fat (scientifically known as *visceral fat*) sits inside your abdominal cavity and wraps around your organs. Belly fat differs from the innocuous type of *subcutaneous fat*, the jiggly fat that is aesthetically unappealing but isn't associated with major disease. On the other hand, studies have shown that excess belly fat promotes disease, because belly fat cells do more than simply store excess calories. These fat cells secrete hormones and inflammatory substances that are linked to a higher risk of type 2 diabetes, insulin resistance, heart disease, and even certain cancers.

Belly fat is very metabolically active compared to subcutaneous fat cells. Belly fat cells release inflammatory substances and free fatty acids into the bloodstream that make a beeline to the liver via the portal vein. (The portal vein carries blood from the intestines, pancreas, and spleen to the liver.) Over time, fat builds up in the liver leading to long-lasting inflammation. Inflammation is the root cause for many of the chronic diseases that plague the human population.

One of the miraculous health benefits of sticking to an intermittent fasting plan is the fact that you can shed *both* subcutaneous fat (just under the skin) and the dangerous belly fat in the abdominal cavity. (Intermittent fasting causes a significant fat cell shrinkage.) In fact, a large review of studies conducted by the Department of Medicine at the University of Illinois at Chicago found that belly fat was reduced by a whopping 4 to 7 percent over a period of 1½ to 6 months in people following intermittent fasting plans.

REMEMBER

Intermittent fasting boosts metabolism while helping you eat fewer calories, a combo that targets abdominal fat cells. Adding in a calorie burn from physical activity gives you a synergistic metabolic furnace, resulting in an efficient way to lose weight and belly fat. A program of regular aerobic exercise, such as fast walking, has also been proven to reduce belly fat — even without dieting. Combine a daily walk with your intermittent fasting plan of choice and start today to whittle away that dangerous belly fat.

BURNING STORED FAT

Fat is stored in fat cells (also known as *adipose tissue*) in the form of *triglycerides* (a string of three bound up chains of fatty acids or what I call *triple fats*). To burn the fat stored for energy, your fat cells must first break apart the triple fat into usable components (usable fats are singular chains of free fatty acids). Then the fat cells must unleash the single fatty acid chains from their storage cells into the bloodstream. Breakdown and release of free fatty acids into the bloodstream (termed *lipolysis* and your ultimate goal) requires enzymes called *lipases*. In the fat cell, lipases work to break down the triple fats into their simple usable form, singular chains of free fatty acids.

Five hormones, released from the following organs during fasting, cause the activation of fat burning enzymes:

- *Glucagon* from the pancreas
- *Growth hormone* from the pituitary gland
- *Adrenocorticotropic hormone (ACTH)* from the pituitary gland
- *Epinephrine* (also known as *adrenaline*) from the adrenal gland
- *Thyroid hormone* from the thyroid gland

After the triglycerides are broken down into single fat chains or free fatty acids inside the fat cells, the fatty acids are released from adipose tissue into the bloodstream. The free fatty acids then travel to cells that are hungry (need energy) and are absorbed. Most tissues in the body are able to use free fatty acids directly as fuel.

Once inside the hungry cells, the single fatty acid chains are transported into the *mitochondria* (the engine or powerhouse of the cell) where they're burned for energy in a process called *beta oxidation*.

The fatty acids can also travel in the bloodstream to the liver. During the fasted state, after the fatty acids enter the liver, they're further broken down to make ketones to feed the body.

Discovering the Numerous Health Benefits to the Body

The myriad health conditions simply refraining from eating for short periods of time positively effects is extensive. Read on to see exactly how and why the act of intermittent fasting has such an extraordinarily salutary effect on the body, a truly fascinating phenomenon.

Outlining the diseases/disorders affected

Fast forward to present day and scientists are truly excited about the data — intermittent fasting is proving to be effective at preventing and improving markers of disease, reducing *oxidative stress* (an imbalance between the production of damaging free radicals and the ability of the body to counteract or detoxify their harmful effects through neutralization by antioxidants), and enhancing learning and memory functioning.

A century of laboratory research links the practice of intermittent fasting with the prevention of age-related disease, including tumors, cardiovascular disease, diabetes, and dementia, to name a few. However, much of that research was conducted in animal models, so the evidence that intermittent fasting holds miracle health benefits for humans is still in its infancy. However, intermittent fasting was prominently featured in a recent review article in the *New England Journal of Medicine*, touting the extraordinary power of intermittent fasting to heal.

Figure 6-1 depicts many of the remarkable health benefits derived from following an intermittent fasting plan. The following list touches on many of these benefits in greater detail:

>> **Promotes weight and fat loss:** Intermittent fasting can help you lose weight and belly fat, without having to consciously restrict calories. Intermittent fasting also amplifies enzymatic fat breakdown (lipolysis). Refer to the earlier section, "Seeing how intermittent fasting targets belly fat," for more information.

>> **Reduces insulin resistance:** Intermittent fasting can sensitize cells to insulin, reducing harmful insulin resistance and lowering blood sugar by 3 to 6 percent. Fasting insulin levels have been lowered by 20 to 31 percent with intermittent fasting, all of which protect against type 2 diabetes. Insulin secretion from the pancreas goes up due to an increase and regeneration of the *beta cells* of the pancreas (the cells that produce and secrete insulin).

>> **Regulates blood sugar:** When your blood sugar is constantly high, your insulin levels are constantly high. This leads to type 2 diabetes, which is a huge epidemic. Consistently high blood sugar levels (also known as *hyperglycemia*) cause damage to the insides of the arteries. Hyperglycemia harms the vessels that supply blood to vital organs, which can increase the risk of heart disease and stroke, kidney disease, vision problems, and nerve problems.

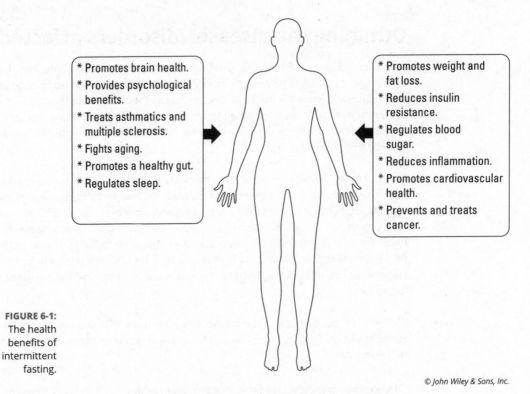

* Promotes brain health.
* Provides psychological benefits.
* Treats asthmatics and multiple sclerosis.
* Fights aging.
* Promotes a healthy gut.
* Regulates sleep.

* Promotes weight and fat loss.
* Reduces insulin resistance.
* Regulates blood sugar.
* Reduces inflammation.
* Promotes cardiovascular health.
* Prevents and treats cancer.

FIGURE 6-1:
The health benefits of intermittent fasting.

© John Wiley & Sons, Inc.

>> **Reduces inflammation:** Research shows that a program of intermittent fasting reduces blood markers of inflammation, a key driver of many chronic diseases. Oxidative stress is one of the factors that accelerates aging and predisposes you to developing disease. Several studies show that intermittent fasting boosts the body's resistance to oxidative stress. Intermittent fasting strengthens immune function and enhances the body's ability to repair cells and DNA.

>> **Promotes cardiovascular health:** Intermittent fasting improves multiple indicators of cardiovascular health in both overweight and normal weight individuals. Intermittent fasting reduces resting heart rate, blood pressure, bad LDL cholesterol, blood triglycerides, inflammation, blood sugar, and insulin resistance — all risk factors for heart disease — the leading cause of death in American men and women. In addition, intermittent fasting lowers inflammation and oxidative stress, both causative factors associated with heart disease.

>> **Prevents and treats cancer:** Some research suggests that intermittent fasting helps fight cancer by lowering insulin resistance and levels of

inflammation. Intermittent fasting may also reverse the effects of chronic conditions such as obesity and type 2 diabetes, which are both risk factors for cancer. Researchers believe that intermittent fasting suppresses tumor growth and extends survival in patients with cancer. Intermittent fasting may make cancer cells more responsive to chemotherapy while protecting other cells. Intermittent fasting also boosts the immune system to help fight cancer that is already present.

» **Promotes brain health:** Intermittent fasting increases production of brain-derived neurotrophic (BDNF), an *anti-aging* protein thought to protect against Alzheimer's disease by helping the brain produce new healthy cells and strengthen existing ones, improving cognition. Intermittent fasting causes the cells in the body to initiate the cellular cleanup process called *autophagy.* (Refer to the section, "Renewing your body with autophagy," later in this chapter for more specifics about how autophagy works in the human body.)

» **Promotes psychological benefits:** Intermittent fasting improves eating behavior and mood. Intermittent fasting increases BDNF, the protein that aids in the growth of new nerve cells. A deficiency of BDNF has been implicated in depression and various other brain problems. BDNF is food for the brain cells, keeping them flourishing, strong, and healthy.

» **Treats asthmatics and multiple sclerosis:** With weight loss comes improvement in asthma symptoms and a reduction in airway resistance. Multiple sclerosis (MS) is an autoimmune disorder characterized by degeneration of the nervous system. Recent studies in people with MS adhering to intermittent fasting programs saw reduced symptoms in as short a period as two months.

» **Fights aging:** Intermittent fasting can extend lifespan in rodents. Studies showed that fasted mice lived 36 to 83 percent longer! Although it's a far cry from mice to men, intermittent fasting has become very popular among the anti-aging crowd. In fact, the health benefits of intermittent fasting on aging, oxidative stress, metabolism, and cardiovascular disease have been demonstrated in both human and animal studies alike.

» **Promotes a healthy gut:** The gut microbiome refers to all the microbes in your intestines, which act as another organ, crucial for your health. More than 1,000 species of bacteria are in the human gut microbiome, and each of them plays a different role in your body. Most of them are extremely important for your health, whereas others may cause disease such inflammatory bowel disease, liver cirrhosis, and colorectal cancer. Scientific research has shown that intermittent fasting restores microbe health and diversity in the gut by increasing the good microbes, augmenting tolerance against bad gut microbes, and rebuilding the integrity of the intestinal wall.

>> **Regulates sleep:** Experts have recommended that adults get about seven to nine hours of sleep per night for good health. Intermittent fasting positively affects your *circadian clock,* which exerts a powerful influence over your sleep. Intermittent fasting strengthens the 24-hour circadian clock. A stronger, more synchronized circadian clock means an easier time falling asleep, staying asleep, and waking feeling refreshed on a regular basis. A good night's sleep will help you function at your best, and to protect your health over time, and with age. (Refer to Chapter 5 for more information about the importance of getting a good night's sleep.)

Considering the mechanics behind the results

Each of the body's systems are positively affected from undergoing repetitive fasted states. The heart, for example, becomes a more efficient machine. Intermittent fasting lowers resting heart rate and blood pressure and promotes a decrease in inflammation and an improvement in resistance to debilitating oxidative stress. Figure 6-2 displays just how intermittent fasting affects each body part.

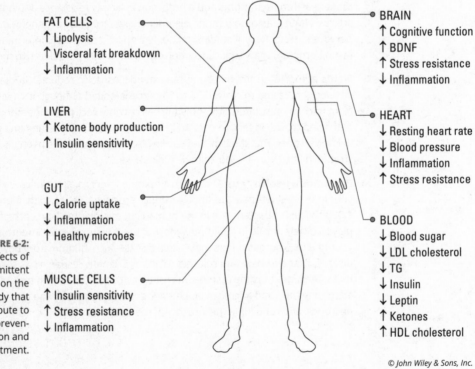

FAT CELLS
↑ Lipolysis
↑ Visceral fat breakdown
↓ Inflammation

LIVER
↑ Ketone body production
↑ Insulin sensitivity

GUT
↓ Calorie uptake
↓ Inflammation
↑ Healthy microbes

MUSCLE CELLS
↑ Insulin sensitivity
↑ Stress resistance
↓ Inflammation

BRAIN
↑ Cognitive function
↑ BDNF
↑ Stress resistance
↓ Inflammation

HEART
↓ Resting heart rate
↓ Blood pressure
↓ Inflammation
↑ Stress resistance

BLOOD
↓ Blood sugar
↓ LDL cholesterol
↓ TG
↓ Insulin
↓ Leptin
↑ Ketones
↑ HDL cholesterol

FIGURE 6-2: Effects of intermittent fasting on the body that contribute to disease prevention and treatment.

© *John Wiley & Sons, Inc.*

Cells can become damaged when they encounter oxidative stress, so preventing or repairing cell damage from oxidative stress is helpful against aging. This stress happens when there is higher-than-normal production of *free radicals* (unstable molecules that carry highly reactive electrons). When free radicals encounter other molecules, a rapid chain reaction occurs forming more and more damaging free radicals. Oftentimes, this process occurs in faulty *mitochondria* (the energy production centers of the cells). Excessive free radical chain reactions cause stress and damage to cellular membranes, essential proteins, and DNA, accelerating aging and promoting disease.

The onslaught of free radicals *is* oxidative stress, the detrimental condition arising from the imbalance between harmful oxidants species and antioxidant defenses. Intermittent fasting boosts internal production of natural free radical–stabilizing antioxidants. The metabolic switch causes cells to turn on survival processes to remove the unhealthy mitochondria and replace them with healthy ones, thus reducing the production of free radicals in the long term. The fasting state also programs cells to cope better with more severe stresses that may come in the future.

Realizing the positive effects on the brain

Intermittent fasting heightens the senses, memory, and ability to learn, sharpening cognitive skills. Fasting gets rid of *brain fog* (a lack of mental clarity) by improving your ability to focus and improving memory. The increase in BDNF observed with intermittent fasting protects your brain from stress and slows brain aging.

Intermittent fasting triggers a dramatic switch in the body's metabolism, flipping the metabolic switch — the state where the body switches fuel from blood sugar to ketones (fat). The use of ketones to feed the hungry brain might help explain several mysteries surrounding brain benefits. From an evolutionary perspective, the brain power that intermittent fasting generates makes sense. Humankind's ancestors typically went days without food, often hunting on an empty stomach. This period of semi-starvation resulted in a brain adaptation, allowing the brain to live off its less preferred fuel, ketones. The use of ketones for brain fuel enhanced cognitive ability and energy so humans would be more likely to obtain food and live another day.

Identifying the benefits for longevity

In today's world, the relationship with food is different than at any other time in human history. Humans evolved over many thousands of years with food as a scarce resource. Today, for many people, the problem isn't food scarcity, but food overabundance — a situation that poses a serious threat to health. High calorie food is everywhere combined with extensive marketing geared toward getting people to eat more. The result? An epidemic of type 2 diabetes and heart disease — chronic illnesses that shorten a person's life span — and are inextricably linked to a person's eating habits and automated, sedentary lifestyle.

After nearly a century of research investigating the effect of calorie restriction on lifespan in animals, the jury is in. Intermittent fasting robustly increases life span. One of the earlier studies on rats placed on a program of alternate day fasting (ADF), which I describe in Chapter 11, showed the average life span of rats increased by up to 80 percent.

Whether intermittent fasting has a similar life-extending effect in humans has yet to be proven. However, many effects of intermittent fasting appear to contribute to a longer life such as a reduction in unhealthful inflammation and a boost in the body's ability to protect itself against oxidative stress, a major contributor to aging and disease.

Renewing your body with autophagy

Perhaps you may have heard all the buzz about this term, *autophagy*, known by some as the cell regenerative diet. In fact, Yoshinori Ohsumi, a Japanese cell biologist, was awarded the Nobel Prize in Physiology or Medicine in 2016 for his discoveries of mechanisms for autophagy. Autophagy is Greek for *self-eating*, which is accurate: Your system ingests the old or damaged proteins and mitochondria and replaces them with brand new ones. So, autophagy is like spring cleaning in your cells.

Intermittent fasting causes extreme autophagy in your body's cells. Autophagy makes your cells younger and more powerful and bolsters antioxidant defenses and DNA repair, which slows aging. The autophagy process not only refers to your body's ability to recycle damaged cells, but also, in some cases, kills cells that no longer serve a purpose. The igniting of autophagy has been linked with promotion of a longer life span. These pathways are untapped in sedentary, overweight people — believed to be one of the many reasons why obesity shortens life span.

With intermittent fasting — during the fasting period — the cells enter autophagy, the stress-resistance mode. Cells are regenerated, damaged molecules are recycled, and all the maintenance and repair work is performed promoting cell survival — all of which support improvements in increased longevity.

Chapter **7**

Determining Whether Intermittent Fasting Is Right for You

What you may not realize is that you're already practicing a form of intermittent fasting. Every night you go to sleep, you're technically fasting. That's why breakfast is called breakfast or *break the fast*. With certain styles of intermittent fasting, you simply extend your nighttime fast longer, which is one reason intermittent fasting is generally safe for most people.

For the vast majority of people who are healthy, without medical issues, intermittent fasting is a safe and superbly healthy lifestyle. However, several subsets of people shouldn't fast. This chapter discusses those people, their conditions, and the reasons why intermittent fasting could be downright dangerous for these people. As you read through these next pages, continuously ask yourself whether intermittent fasting is the right fit for you.

If you want to start with an intermittent fasting plan, check out the Cheat Sheet at www.dummies.com by searching for "Intermittent Fasting For Dummies Cheat Sheet" to find a quick list of ten tips to remember before you begin a plan.

Getting Permission from Your Personal Doctor

Seeing your doctor for regular health exams and tests is essential for preventive medicine purposes. Annual physicals also can help find problems early, when your chances for treatment and cure are better. Unfortunately, the current healthcare system isn't truly a healthcare system. The United States has a medical (that is, sick) care organization — a practice that waits until people become ill before it kicks into action — instead of a healthcare system focused on helping Americans prevent disease and stay healthy.

You can get ahead of the game and take your health into your own hands by scheduling all the preventive tests, screenings, and doctor visits required for your age and gender. Doing so can help your chances for living a longer, healthier life.

WARNING

If you're seeing your personal physician for a specific health issue, then you must review with her the type of intermittent fasting you intend to follow and get her permission. Some people should be extra cautious; I discuss who should pay special attention to following an intermittent fasting plan in the section, "Recognizing Who Shouldn't Intermittent Fast" later in this chapter. If you have a medical condition, you must consult with your doctor before trying intermittent fasting.

You can begin to assess your own health status by tuning in to your numbers, the easy way to see in black and white where you are health-wise and where you need to go. This section gauges whether an intermittent fasting lifestyle is going to work for you.

Know your numbers

Even if you consider yourself healthy, I still suggest you run your intermittent fasting program by your personal physician before you start. During this appointment you can discuss the pros and cons of beginning your intermittent fasting journey, and she can take your vital signs. This information will allow her to monitor the myriad health change that will occur during your new lifestyle.

Before you start your intermittent fasting plan, your doctor should administer the following tests:

>> Your weight and height

>> Your heart rate and blood pressure

>> Baseline bloodwork that includes your cholesterol, triglycerides, and fasting blood sugar levels

Table 7-1 shows you what the medical experts consider to be ideal numbers for good health.

TABLE 7-1 **Ideal Test Numbers to Aim For**

Test	Ideal Value
Total cholesterol	Less than 200
LDL cholesterol (the bad kind)	Less than 100
HDL cholesterol (the good kind)	50 and higher
Triglycerides	Less than 150
Fasting blood sugar	Less than 100
Blood pressures	Less than 120/80
Resting heart rate	Less than 80 beats per minute

TIP

Flip to Chapter 23 and access your toolbox and be sure to write all your starting medical numbers in your journal. After your get the go-ahead from your physician, make a follow-up appointment for three to six months, repeat all the tests, and record your new numbers in your journal. The changes you write will motivate you to keep on track with your new, healthy lifestyle.

Give it time

If you get your doctor's approval to try intermittent fasting, consider which plan in Part 3 best fits your lifestyle, and then be sure to create short- and long-term health and fitness goals. (You can find goal worksheets in Chapter 23.)

REMEMBER

Regardless of the plan you choose, proceed slowly. Research has shown that it takes at least a month to adapt to the rigors of intermittent fasting. Most people are used to eating three meals a day plus snacks. Changing this ingrained routine takes time and practice. Most experts believe that slow is better for attaining a sustainable weight loss and health benefits that last. Most people will need to follow the intermittent fasting basic rules for at least ten weeks to witness some positive results.

If, at your follow-up doctor visit, your new numbers haven't changed as much as you had hoped, revisit your options. Here are four actions you can take to boost your intermittent fasting results:

» **Switch to a different plan.** There are multiple intermittent fasting plans, and there is no one-size-fits-all. For instance, if you didn't see results on the 16:8 plan, then try switching it to perhaps the Warrior plan.

» **Eat less during your eating windows.** The most common reason people don't have success on their intermittent fasting journey is that they eat anything and everything during their eating windows. Now is a good time to tap into your emergency backup system; flip to Chapter 3 and do the calorie calculations.

» **Eat healthier foods during your eating window.** Just because intermittent fasting focuses on when you eat rather than what you eat doesn't give you the green light to engage in a junk food free-for-all eat fest. Consuming sugar-, fat-, and salt-laden processed foods will negate many of the fasting-derived health benefits. Try making the following Mediterranean-style nutritious foods a priority in your diet:

  ● **Healthy fats:** Extra-virgin olive oil, nuts, and avocado

  ● **Lean proteins:** Beans, fish, and skinless poultry

  ● **Good carbohydrates:** 100 percent whole grains

  ● **Fiber and antioxidant-filled foods:** Fruits and vegetables

» **Drink enough calorie-free beverages during your fasting windows:** Fasting or not, staying hydrated helps you fight off hunger and cravings by helping you to feel full. During the fasted state, the body is breaking down and recycling waste. Your body needs water to detoxify and flush out the toxins, so drink up!

TIP

Intermittent fasting may not be for everybody, but there is no doubt that eating healthier is the key to health for everybody. If you need some help, focus on eating the plant-based Mediterranean way in Chapter 17 — the healthiest diet for disease prevention and longevity.

Throwing a Big Red Flag — Warnings for Diabetics

Studies on the safety and benefits of intermittent fasting with diabetes are limited. That being said, if you're diabetic and you're considering intermittent fasting, don't do it on your own. Do it only under the close supervision of your healthcare provider and with appropriate personal glucose monitoring.

If you have your blood sugar under control (fasting number under 100) and your doctor hasn't diagnosed you with diabetes or pre-diabetes (fasting blood sugar between 100 to 125), then feel free to skip this section. Here I shed some light on the disease that is epidemic around the globe.

Assessing type 1 and type 2 diabetes

There are two main types of diabetes: type 1 and type 2. Both types of diabetes are chronic diseases that affect the way your body regulates blood sugar.

Type 2 is by far the most common type of diabetes in the United States. (According to the Centers for Disease Control and Prevention [CDC], 90 to 95 percent of people with diabetes in the United States have type 2. Just 5 percent of people have type 1.) Table 7-2 compares the two types of diabetes.

TABLE 7-2   **Comparing Type 1 and Type 2 Diabetes**

Type 1 Diabetes	Type 2 Diabetes
Autoimmune disease.	Metabolic condition.
Immune system attacks the beta cells of the pancreas.	The pancreas no longer produces enough insulin or the cells are resistant to insulin.
The pancreas can no longer produce insulin.	The pancreas still functions, just not efficiently.
The pancreas produces *no* insulin.	The pancreas usually produces some insulin, but either the amount produced isn't enough for the body's needs or the body's cells are resistant to it.
Treatment requires insulin injections and constant glucose monitoring.	Treatment involves diet, exercise, oral medications, and eventually insulin.
Risk factors include genetics and environmental factors.	Risk factors include genetics and being overweight and sedentary.
Complications include the following:	Complications include the following:
Cardiovascular disease, including a risk of heart attack and stroke Kidney disease and kidney failure	Cardiovascular disease, including a risk of heart attack and stroke
	Kidney disease and kidney failure
Eye problems and vision loss	Eye problems and vision loss
Nerve damage	Nerve damage
Problems with wound healing which could lead to amputations	Problems with wound healing which could lead to amputations
Ketoacidosis	

The benefits of type 1 diabetics following a program of intermittent fasting differ from those observed in type 2 diabetics. Most type 1 diabetics aren't overweight. However, they're at great risk of cardiovascular disease. Intermittent fasting has been proven to reduce risk of developing heart disease, which would be beneficial for type 1 diabetics. Intermittent fasting is a catalyst for numerous potential health benefits and can be carried out safely in patients with type 1 diabetes with the guidance of an experienced healthcare provider.

WARNING

Type 1 diabetes does require close consultation with your physician and blood sugar monitoring. The risk of hypoglycemia with fasting in type 1 diabetics is extremely risky. Talk to your doctor first. If you have type 1 diabetes or have had hypoglycemia, your doctor may recommend you not fast.

The benefits of intermittent fasting for type 2 diabetics are multi-fold. Insulin resistance (and associated inflammation) and obesity are the most prominent features of type 2 diabetes as is accumulation of visceral (belly) fat. In type 2 diabetes, the body becomes less sensitive to insulin and the resulting insulin resistance also leads to chronic inflammation.

Intermittent fasting programs have been proven to promote insulin sensitivity, reduce insulin levels, and fight inflammation. By making cells more sensitive to insulin, fasting blood sugar levels will dramatically drop. Furthermore, high levels of insulin trigger accumulation of fat around the belly and on major organs in the abdomen. The fat cells produce chemicals that lead to inflammation. Reducing blood insulin levels and losing belly fat tames the inflammation and helps reverse the hallmarks of this deadly disease.

Also, intermittent fasting is effective at helping people lose weight and melt away belly fat — both common adverse health conditions associated with type 2 diabetes. Intermittent fasting markedly reverses various metabolic and inflammatory pathways that plague type 2 diabetics. Recent studies have shown that programs of intermittent fasting dramatically improve fasting blood sugar levels and promote weight loss in people with type 2 diabetes.

Focusing on the risks

Intermittent fasting does have some potential risks for diabetics. Those risks include the following:

>> **Hypoglycemia:** The most immediate risk with intermittent fasting is the potential for *hypoglycemia* (low blood sugar) in diabetics, a condition that can be life-threatening. Both types of diabetics take some form of antidiabetic

medications that are associated with hypoglycemia, specifically insulin and *sulfonylureas* (oral medications prescribed for type 2 diabetes).

Discuss with your physician preventive and treatment measures for hypoglycemic attacks. Doses of antidiabetic medications should be adjusted on days of intermittent fasting. Most important, the goal with diabetes is to maintain a steady and stable blood sugar throughout the day, so work with your healthcare provider to prevent those highs and lows in blood sugar.

» **Ketoacidosis:** *Diabetic ketoacidosis* is a complication of type 1 diabetes. This life-threatening condition results from dangerously high levels of ketones and sugar in the bloodstream. Ketoacidosis occurs when the body can't produce enough insulin (insulin brings blood sugar into the cells). When the body doesn't have enough insulin, the body overproduces ketones. The *ketones* (a chemical your body produces when it burns stored fat too quickly) build up in the system. This combination of high amounts of sugar and ketones makes the blood too acidic, which can lead to a diabetic coma or death.

Ketosis is the presence of ketones in the blood and is not harmful. Ketosis differs from ketoacidosis. I discuss ketosis in greater detail in Chapter 5.

Recognizing Who Shouldn't Intermittent Fast

Intermittent fasting can have its drawbacks. The beginning weeks of intermittent fasting usually have the most issues. Periods of fasting at the start may be accompanied by fatigue, irritability, or dizziness, because the body needs time to get used to utilizing ketones for energy instead of glucose.

WARNING

You should *not* practice intermittent fasting if

» **You're underweight or have an eating disorder.** Underweight is classified as having a Body Mass Index (BMI) lower than 18.5 (refer to Chapter 2 to help you determine your BMI). If your BMI is low or you have an eating disorder like anorexia, you need the calories and eating disorders can be deadly. (Refer to the next section for more about eating disorders.)

» **You're pregnant.** You need extra nutrients and calories to support growth and development of your child.

» **You're breastfeeding.** You need extra nutrients and calories for your child and to keep your milk supply intact.

During a fasted state, pregnant or breastfeeding women may run out of glucose and burn fat, but also, due to their revved-up metabolisms, resort to burning tissue and muscle for energy. Furthermore, if a pregnant woman overproduces ketones, the effect can be harmful to the fetus.

>> **You're trying to conceive.** Following a high nutrient diet before you conceive will boost your fertility and lower the risk of birth defects.

>> **You have a history of amenorrhea.** *Amenorrhea* is a cessation of menstruation. You need the calories to prevent menstrual disorders.

>> **You have thyroid hormone issues.** Following intermittent fasting may interfere with thyroid hormone production, which can be especially harmful if you have autoimmune issues.

>> **You have hormone balance issues.** Excessive restriction of calories may exacerbate a disruption of hormone balance. Such disturbances can cause menstrual cycle disorders in women and reduced testosterone in men.

>> **You're younger than 18.** Children need extra nutrients to grow. Check out the section, "Restricting Children from Intermittent Fasting," later in this chapter for more information.

>> **You're an elite athlete and perform high levels of physical activity.** Given that high-level athletes require much more nutrition than non-elite athletes and many have trouble getting in enough calories to fuel their sport, intermittent fasting isn't recommended.

>> **You're a senior with an unsteady gait.** In the elderly, fluctuations in blood sugar concentration can cause instability of the body, which can result in an increased number of falls, and even fractures due to osteoporosis.

If you meet any of the following, you may be able to fast, but only with medical supervision:

>> If you have type 1 or type 2 diabetes mellitus

>> If you take *any* prescription medications

>> If you have *any* serious medical conditions such as cancer, liver disease, kidney disease, or heart disease

Other risks of fasting, in general, include a variety of potential harms related to insufficient calorie intake and some due to dehydration. Adverse events may include dizziness, nausea, insomnia, falls, migraine headache, weakness that limits daily activities, and excessive hunger pangs. The presence of a chronic disease can exacerbate the risk of experiencing many of these side effects. For people with chronic diseases, make sure you get permission from your physician before you start any intermittent fasting plan. After you start, ensure your physician monitors you. Refer to the section, "Getting Permission from Your Personal Doctor," earlier in this chapter for why it's important.

REMEMBER

Like the warning labels on OTC drugs, the potential side effects of intermittent fasting that I outline in this chapter are numerous and can be unsettling for some people. However, most people following an intermittent fasting plan don't experience any side effects except, perhaps, hunger pangs. Flip to Chapter 15 to address the most common potential speed bumps you may face and how you can overcome them.

Surveying the Eating Disorder Silent Epidemic

Eating disorders are complex mental health conditions that often require the intervention of medical and psychological experts to alter their course. Experts have termed eating disorders a silent epidemic, with at least 30 million Americans afflicted, according to the National Association of Anorexia Nervosa and Associated Disorders (ANAD).

They're silent, because individuals who have eating disorders tend to be secretive about them. They are often ashamed of their illness or want to hide it. Only 10 percent of individuals with eating disorders seek and receive treatment, according to the ANAD. The *American Journal of Psychiatry* notes that eating disorders have the highest mortality rate of any mental illness. And, based on ANAD statistics, about a million Americans will die from an eating disorder. Anyone with an eating disorder shouldn't go on an intermittent fasting program.

The three most common eating disorders are as follows:

>> **Binge-eating disorder:** This disorder is out-of-control eating that shames sufferers and stresses organ function; it's three times more prevalent than anorexia and bulimia combined, affecting approximately 15 million Americans and slightly more females than males.

>> **Bulimia:** People with bulimia compulsively binge on large amounts of food and then attempt to purge the calories through compensatory behaviors like vomiting, using laxatives, using of diet pills, and exercising. Bulimia affects approximate 4.7 million females and 1.5 million males.

> » **Anorexia nervosa:** *Anorexia* is starvation characterized by food restriction or compulsive exercise that triggers medically perilous weight loss. It's the second deadliest mental illness after opioid addiction. Anorexia affects about 1 percent of females, and 0.3 percent of males.

WEB EXTRAS

If you think a friend or loved one has an eating disorder, steer her or him toward professional treatment before the situation worsens. Contact the National Eating Disorders Association at www.nationaleatingdisorders.org/.

Restricting Children from Intermittent Fasting

Childhood overweight and obesity is of epidemic proportions in the United States, afflicting more than 30 percent of children, making it the most common chronic disease of childhood. Childhood obesity isn't just a cosmetic problem; it's a real health problem that can be associated with significant health issues in childhood and in adulthood. If you're a parent of overweight young children, you should actively seek help to determine why your child is overweight and act with your pediatrician to help rectify the situation.

WARNING

What you must *not* do is place your child on a program of intermittent fasting. Here's why:

> » Children are developing, their cerebrums are developing, their muscles are developing. Low calorie intake could hinder growth.

> » Children need all the calories available to them to keep them alert and attentive at school and throughout the day.

> » What works for adults may not be best for kids. Children have their own set of nutritional needs for healthy growth and development.

The safest way to help overweight children lose weight is to work with a registered dietitian and pediatrician.

3
Evaluating the Most Popular Intermittent Fasting Plans

Discover the rules of the road: what to eat during your feasting periods and what is allowed during your fasting periods.

Examine the five most popular methods of practicing intermittent fasting.

Look closer at each of these intermittent fasting variations for examples and sample schedules.

Identify the positives and negatives of each intermittent fasting plan.

Compare and contrast each method so you can discover which intermittent fasting eating pattern best fits into your schedule and is the most viable strategy for you.

Chapter **8**

Knowing What to Eat During Your Fasting and Feasting Times

You're ready to begin your fasting journey, but before you start let me give you guidance on what types of food to eat to complement and maximize the results of the intermittent fast you choose to follow. Before I delve into what to eat and what not to eat, I give you some encouragement to help you get into the right mind-set and clarify your fasting and feasting goals. I then examine in plain English just what you need to know about what to eat, what not to eat, and why.

Keeping Your Goals

Chapter 2 provides advice about setting your goals when incorporating an intermittent fasting plan in your life. As you move forward in your journey, keep the two goals in this section front and center.

Fasting goal — Deplete your glucose stores

Fast the right way to get to your golden *fasted state* that occurs when the body has depleted all its glucose (blood sugar) stores. Shifting into the fat-burning state, known as *ketosis*, occurs after you've burned through your *glycogen stores* (the carbs stored in your muscles and liver). That's when the metabolic switch occurs and alternative sources of energy (fat) can be metabolized and used as fuel (in the form of ketones).

REMEMBER

To ensure that you don't confuse your body and prevent attaining this ketotic state, *you can't consume any significant source of calories during your fast.* If you consume calories, regardless of the source (carbs, fat, or protein), your pancreas releases insulin and the metabolic switch is turned off. Protein requires insulin for metabolism, as do carbohydrate and fats. Refer to Chapter 5 for more about the science behind intermittent fasting and what you want to achieve during your short-term fasted states.

Feasting goal — Consume healthful foods

When your feasting time arrives, eat a healthful, plant-based Mediterranean diet. Don't fall for the garbage advice to follow a high-protein, low-carb diet. If followed for the long term, these diets have been proven to promote diseases such as diabetes, colon cancer, and cardiovascular disease. Stick to what the nutrition scientists who have researched the healthiest way to eat for decades say. Hands down, the results are a plant-based, whole foods, Mediterranean diet. Refer to the section, "Seeing why eating Mediterranean is smart," later in this chapter for more about the Mediterranean diet. To see the plethora of health benefits you'll experience from intermittent fasting, check out Chapter 6. Combine the two diet strategies to achieve optimal health.

What You Can Eat When You're Fasting

Your fasting window has arrived, now what? Hopefully, you've prepared ahead and can reach for your liquids of choice and start drinking. The following sections explain what you can consume during your fasting windows to accelerate your results.

Drinking your way through your intermittent fast

There are plenty of liquids you can put in your mouth to help assuage hunger and keep you healthy and hydrated. Follow the guidelines in Table 8-1 to see what you can drink during your intermittent fast:

TABLE 8-1 **What You Can Drink during Fasting Periods**

Yes	No
Do drink plain old water (and lots of it).	Don't add calorie-containing flavorings.
Do drink unflavored, calorie-free sparkling water, seltzer water, mineral water, and zero calorie-flavored waters.	Don't drink waters with calories.
Do drink black coffee (either caffeinated or decaffeinated). The next section provides more info.	Don't add *anything* except a calorie-free sweetener (if so desired).
Do drink brewed or herbal tea (no additives).	Don't add anything except a calorie-free sweetener (if so desired). Tea must be brewed and sugar-free. Add a calorie-free sweetener (if desired).
Do drink diet drinks.	Don't drink sodas — any canned or bottled beverages with calories.
Do chew zero calorie sugar free gum (if so desired).	Don't chew regular gum or mints.

REMEMBER You may be surprised to see that artificial sweeteners are allowed during your fasting periods. This topic is quite controversial; however, the science is irrefutable. A recent meta-analysis published in the *European Journal of Clinical Nutrition* reported that consuming non-nutritive sweeteners does *not* raise blood sugar level.

Furthermore, some people believe that artificial sweeteners don't satisfy the biological sugar cravings in the same manner as sugar and can lead to increased food intake. This hasn't been proven. In fact, replacing sugar with artificial sweeteners has been shown to help people lose weight.

Splenda and stevia are popular types of virtually calorie-free sweeteners. Although no scientific evidence suggests that either is unsafe, it appears that stevia (derived from a plant rather than in the lab) is associated with the fewest concerns. Like all foods, consume these sweeteners in moderation. Fasting is hard, and if the use of artificial sweeteners is helpful to you in getting you through your fasting periods, then by all means use them!

Loving black coffee

Black coffee is the best nutrition news to come along since dark chocolate became the new health food. Coffee has long been a subject of debate over whether it's beneficial or harmful for health. If you're a coffee lover, you can rejoice because recent studies have established that coffee is indeed a healthy drink. Of course, you need to control the quantity and also nix the additives to truly enjoy its health benefits.

What about the caffeine in coffee? To give you some perspective: The average amount of caffeine in a standard 8-ounce cup of brewed coffee is between 80 to 135 mg, whereas an 8-ounce cup of green tea has only about 15 mg. A handful of dark chocolate–covered coffee espresso beans (28 beans) contain 336 mg of caffeine. Four roasted espresso beans contain 24 mg of caffeine, the approximate amount in a 6-ounce cup of brewed tea.

The following sections take a closer look at the many health benefits to drinking coffee:

Examining the health benefits to coffee

Recent research has linked coffee with many numerous health benefits, and you can safely drink up to eight 8-ounce cups a day. Here are some of the findings:

>> **Increased longevity:** A large study, published in the journal *JAMA*, of a half million people, found that those people drinking from one to eight cups of coffee per day lived longer than people who abstained from drinking coffee altogether. Note that this was an observational study that only shows an association and doesn't prove cause and effect.

>> **Reduced heart disease and stroke risk:** Good news connecting coffee drinking with prevention of cardiovascular disease from scientists presenting findings at an American Heart Association conference. The researchers analyzed data from the long-running Framingham Heart Study, which includes information about what people eat and their cardiovascular health. They found that drinking coffee was associated with decreased risk of developing heart failure by 7 percent and stroke by 8 percent with every additional cup of coffee consumed per week compared with non-coffee drinkers.

>> **Reduced risk of type 2 diabetes:** A review study published in the journal *Diabetology and Metabolic Syndrome* concluded that frequent coffee drinkers have a substantially lower risk of developing type 2 diabetes mellitus. Moderate coffee intake (equal to or less than four cups of coffee per day) is the dose most associated with a decrease in the risk of type 2 diabetes. Scientists surmise that the antioxidant level in coffee improves insulin sensitivity that eventually helps in lowering the risk of type 2 diabetes.

>> **Reduced risk of gallstones:** Research finding published in the *British Medical Journal* found that men who drink two to three cups of coffee a day have a 4 percent lower risk of developing gallstones than those who don't drink coffee regularly, and men who drink four or more cups a day have a 45 percent lower risk.

>> **Reduced risk of neurodegenerative conditions such as Alzheimer's and Parkinson's diseases:** Some recent research has supported the role of coffee consumption in decreasing the risk of Alzheimer's and Parkinson's disease. A study published in the journal *Frontiers in Neuroscience* found that coffee consumption, especially dark roast coffee, interferes with the production of the toxic misfolded protein masses, called *amyloid plaques,* the hallmark of dementia.

Additional studies have linked coffee consumption with other health benefits, including:

>> **Increased fat loss:** A recent study published in the *Journal of Nutrition* found that women who drink two or three cups of coffee a day have lower total body and abdominal fat than those who drink less. Nutritionists also recommend coffee for its low-calorie content.

>> **Mood elevation:** Coffee also elevates your mood, a phenomenon that is more related to the caffeine in coffee. Caffeine is a plant chemical (alkaloid) that is found in many foods and beverages such as coffee, tea, chocolate, some types of soda, energy drinks, and sports products. In fact, caffeine is legally classified as a drug and is the most popular drug in the United States. Caffeine boosts your alertness and elevates your mood by blocking the action of one brain chemical (*adenosine*) while simultaneously boosting production of another (*serotonin*). Serotonin is that feel-good hormone that is significantly increased after eating chocolate, for example.

>> **Energy boost:** Caffeine acts as a stimulant for the central nervous system, it increases heart rate and blood pressure, and boosts the release of adrenaline from the adrenal glands. A person's response to caffeine is individualized with many individuals developing a tolerance to the effects of caffeine; therefore, they aren't affected by the potential side effects: jitteriness, nervousness, upset stomach, and sleeplessness.

CAFFEINE ISN'T FOR EVERYONE

People experience different effects when consuming caffeine, and they may have different levels of tolerance to it. For people with a caffeine sensitivity, consuming low amounts may lead to symptoms such as nausea, anxiety, restlessness, and insomnia. If you're sensitive to caffeine, you should drink decaf so you can still benefit from the antioxidant boost, without the jitters.

>> **Antioxidant boost:** A cup of java can do more than just give you that morning wake-up call. In fact, coffee beans top the list for Americans' source of antioxidants. Antioxidants help the body fight off disease by scavenging up dangerous free radicals. *Free radicals* are harmful terrorist-type by-products of metabolism and contribute to the development of numerous chronic diseases such as cancer and heart disease. Bumping up your antioxidant intake will help your body dismantle the free radicals and ward off disease. The large amount of antioxidants in coffee will reduce inflammation and your risk of disease.

Seeing how coffee can help you succeed during your fast

Drinking black coffee can help you during your fasts and is an immensely helpful tool. Black coffee

>> Dulls your hunger

>> Boosts your perceived energy level

>> Helps get you through your fast

When you drink your coffee black, you can taste its real flavor, and when you get used to it, there's no turning back! I encourage you to explore the different taste nuances of coffee. You'll discover coffee is filled with unique flavors that can delight your senses. Cream and sugar dull those flavors so you don't even know they are there, which is why every coffee lover should drink black coffee. Not to mention, drinking black coffee is extremely convenient. You can grab a cup of black coffee almost anywhere without worrying if they have your favorite additives.

TIP

Coffee is totally optional and not necessary for intermittent fasting. If coffee is out, drink tea, especially black and green teas — proven to be health-boosting bonanzas as well.

What You Can Eat When You're Feasting

You have a choice about the kinds of foods you'll eat during your feasting periods. I suggest you do the smarter combo — what I call the "InterMediterranean fasting plan." Feed yourself well and your body will respond. By adding in the superbly healthy plant-based, Mediterranean style of eating combined with your selected style of intermittent fasting, you create a formidable disease-prevention and anti-aging lifestyle. You can't deny the health benefits of the Mediterranean Diet, and the fact the food tastes so delicious is a major bonus. Chapter 17 gives you the lowdown on the Mediterranean Diet. Here I touch on the types of foods you should be ingesting during your eating windows to maximize your intermittent fasting outcomes.

Knowing what to eat: Some quick tips

By aiming to fill your meals with nutrient-dense, portion-controlled amounts of food (including slow, complex carbs to prevent blood sugar swings during your fast) like you'll eat on a plant-based diet, you'll have more energy and better results from your program.

Here are some quick tips to follow during your eating window:

>> Snack on healthy foods such as a handful of nuts, some fresh fruit with non-fat Greek yogurt, an apple with some peanut butter, or fresh veggies dipped in hummus.

>> Don't drink your calories unless it's a glass of red wine with your meal. Gulping down sugar-laden soft drinks or sweetened juices or iced teas makes it simple to swallow gargantuan amounts of calories in minutes.

>> Balance your meals with a whole grain, lean protein (mostly plant protein), lots of deeply colored veggies, extra virgin olive oil, and seasoned with salt alternatives such as citrus, garlic, vinegars, fresh herbs, and spices.

The combination of high-nutrient foods will give you the energy you need to enhance the benefits of your intermittent fasting journey.

Why eating a plant-based diet is smart

Diet plays a huge role in the prevention of cardiovascular diseases — the leading cause of death in American men and women. The foods typically eaten when following a whole food, plant-based contain a plethora of Mother Nature's natural disease-prevention medicine. These substances, to name just a few, are

>> **Polyphenols:** *Polyphenols* are plant chemicals that when consumed frequently can boost digestion and brain health as well as protect against heart disease, type 2 diabetes, and even certain cancers. Polyphenols are naturally found in plant foods, such as fruits, vegetables, herbs, spices, tea, dark chocolate, and wine. Powerful antioxidants, they can neutralize dangerous free radicals as well as reduce inflammation, which is the key driver of many chronic diseases.

>> **Resveratrol:** Another nutraceutical found in foods of the plant kingdom deserving specific consideration is *resveratrol.* Dark red and purple grapes are rich in resveratrol, which is why the largest concentration is found in red wine, but resveratrol is also found in blueberries, peanuts, and pistachios. The antioxidant properties of resveratrol are well established and are responsible for its heart-protection actions and ability to improve blood pressure. Furthermore, resveratrol increases adiponectin concentrations (*adiponectin* is a hormone with a healthful anti-inflammatory effect).

>> **Carotenoids:** *Carotenoids* are plant pigments responsible for the bright red, yellow, and orange hues found in many fruits and vegetables. They're present in high concentration in carrots, tomatoes, pumpkin, nectarines, papaya, and also in seaweed. Their beneficial effect in preventing heart attacks is attributed to antioxidant and anti-inflammatory functions.

Weighing Keto and Intermittent Fasting — Not a Healthy Combination

Intermittent fasting focuses on when you eat rather than what you eat, so you choose the type of diet to accompany your intermittent fasting plan. I suggest you *avoid* choosing the Keto Diet as your combo eating plan of choice, which may be confusing for you because a lot of chatter on the Internet touts the purported dream combination of keto and fasting. People who combine keto and intermittent fasting use the regimen to further push their body into ketosis. Here I discuss in more depth why you shouldn't follow the Keto Diet and intermittent fasting together and how the allowable and forbidden foods don't mesh.

Understanding why the Keto Diet and intermittent fasting don't mix

Here is why you shouldn't use the Keto Diet as your intermittent fasting diet of choice:

» **Dieters going keto tend to lose weight, but the wrong way**. The Keto Diet is low in fiber and high in saturated fat, which is a risk for cardiovascular disease. Many followers eat a meat-centric diet, with excessive intake of red and processed meats — proven to increase the risk for dying from heart disease, according to research published in the journal *Nutrients*. Furthermore, the Keto Diet can harm the gut microbe, an important part of your metabolic health. Take it from me, a credentialed nutrition scientist, following a Keto Diet is *not* healthy!

» **Ketosis for long periods is unsafe.** Ignore the hype, and don't buy into the attraction of eating to promote further *ketosis* (the process that occurs when your body doesn't have enough carbs to burn for energy). Instead, the body burns fat and makes things called ketones, which it can use for fuel. (Note that *ketoacidosis* is a higher level of ketones in the body compared to ketosis, occurs in diabetics and is life-threatening.) Refer to Chapter 7 for an extensive discussion on diabetes. Safe and effective intermittent fasting puts your body into ketosis for short time periods followed by feeding your body with the nutrients it needs to prevent disease whereas the Keto Diet puts your body into ketosis, but it's unhealthy because it's seriously restrictive, cuts out super nutritious foods, and is hard to follow.

REMEMBER

The fasting phase puts your body into ketosis, *not* the diet. Granted, the allure of intermittent fasting is that *you* choose what you eat and when you eat. However, to double up on the health and fitness benefits of your intermittent fasting journey, choose your eating plan wisely.

» **The Keto Diet is missing key nutrients.** The Keto Diet is a trendy high-fat, low-carb meal plan that is simply a recycled age-old, super high-fat, high-protein, and ultra-low carb diet packaged into a new, highly attractive, and immensely popular fad eating plan. The foods promoted are especially high in dangerous bad fats and animal protein. In fact, the diet requires roughly 80 percent of your daily calories to come from fat, much of it considered bad fat (see the next section for some examples). The harmful heart-health repercussions of following this diet long term haven't been revealed. Many of the foods that the diet plan excludes are the main source of disease-preventing and free radical–halting antioxidants.

What's wrong about keto: What you shouldn't and should be eating

The Keto Diet is ridiculously heavy in red meat and other fatty, processed, and salty foods that are notoriously disease-promoting. So many of the recommended foods in this diet simply aren't what your body needs to maintain and promote good health.

Here are the foods often suggested on the Keto Diet that you should *not* eat and substitutions for healthier living:

>> **Coconut oil:** It's high is artery-clogging saturated fatty acids. You should use extra-virgin olive oil (EVOO) as your main fat and occasionally canola oil in lieu of coconut oil.

>> **Red and processed meats:** They're high in dietary cholesterol and saturated fats. Red and processed meat consumption is associated with increased mortality and colon cancer. Switch to lean seafood and plant proteins as your main sources of lean protein.

>> **Full-fat cheeses:** These types of cheeses are high in dietary cholesterol and saturated fats. Switch to reduced fat cheeses and small amounts of strong, flavorful full fat cheese as a garnish.

>> **Full-fat dairy (milk):** Full-fat dairy is high in dietary cholesterol and saturated fats. Switch to fat-free milk or plant milk alternatives.

The following foods are forbidden on the Keto Diet, but they're the exact foods you *should* be eating:

>> **Beans, peas, lentils, and peanuts:** Legumes are extremely nutritious; in fact, lentil consumption has been associated with longevity. Many studies have found that increasing consumption of antioxidant-packed beans decreases the risk of obesity, diabetes, and overall mortality while promoting increased energy and a lower weight. Additional benefits of beans include strengthening of bones due to the high magnesium content, a mineral which is involved in bone health metabolism. Beans, especially dark beans, are incredibly heart healthy. The fiber, potassium, folate, vitamin B6, and phytonutrient content of beans, coupled with their lack of cholesterol, all support heart health. This unique fiber also lowers the total amount of cholesterol in the blood, especially bad LDL cholesterol, making "beans, beans, good for your heart!". Beans also feed the mighty microbes — the good healthy microbes in our gut promoting disease-prevention.

>> **Grains, such as rice, pasta, and oatmeal:** Yes, the grains should be whole, but excluding these grains — the staff of life — is ludicrous. You need the fiber

and significant amount of nutrition that these carbs provide to maintain and promote a long and healthy life.

>> **Low-fat dairy products:** Dairy products are a nutritious source of calcium and protein for most people. They should be eaten in the fat-free form to extricate artery-clogging saturated fat found in whole dairy foods.

>> **Most fruits, except for lemons, limes, tomatoes, and small portions of berries:** To exclude any fruit is ridiculous. About 90 percent of people don't eat enough fruits and vegetables for good health — one possible contributing cause of the obesity epidemic.

>> **Most alcohols, including wine:** Red wine consumed in moderation is heart-healthy and a cornerstone of the Mediterranean Diet.

>> **Starchy vegetables, including corn, potatoes, and peas:** Starchy vegetables are super nutritious *slow carbs* (plant foods rich in fiber and, therefore, take longer to digest and cause a slower rise in blood sugar) that should be part of a healthy diet and especially an intermittent fasting program. Refer to Table 8-2 for a list of additional healthful slow carbs to include in your diet.

TABLE 8-2

Slow-Digesting Carbs

Fruits	Vegetables	Legumes/Nuts	Whole Grains
Apples	Okra	Beans	Steel cut oats
Oranges	Zucchini	Peas	Quinoa
Peaches	Asparagus	Lentils	Brown rice
Pears	Carrots	Walnuts	Pumpernickel
Plums	Kale	Almonds	Barley
	Cauliflower		
	Parsnips		
	Yams		

REMEMBER

A plant-based whole foods diet like the Mediterranean Diet is the best way to promote health and longevity and is the most effective add-on to your intermittent fasting lifestyle. The intermittent fast and *not the diet* is what activates *metabolic switching* and *cellular stress resistance* — the main triggers for the numerous health benefits that this lifestyle offers. Refer to Chapter 5 for more information about the science of intermittent fasting. Keep in mind, fasting can be difficult at first. Flip to Chapter 6 to peruse the phenomenal health benefits associated with intermittent fasting.

Chapter **9**

Trying the 16:8 Time-Restricted Intermittent Fasting Plan

I ntermittent fasting is an increasingly popular dietary approach used for both weight loss and overall health. The most popular form (and easiest) intermittent fast is called the *time-restricted plan.* I like to think of this form of fasting as the *eating-window diet.* You decide when and for how long you open your window of eating.

Time-restricted intermittent fasting means you limit your eating and fasting periods to a set number of hours every day — hence, the name the eating window. The most common time-restricted pattern is the 16:8 intermittent fast, which is where you eat all your food for the day in an 8-hour period — eat as often as you wish during this window. The remaining 16 hours is your fasting period where no calories are consumed (only calorie-free beverages and lots of water). You repeat this exact pattern daily.

Although there are numerous variations to the time-restricted intermittent fasting plan, this chapter focuses on the 16:8 intermittent fasting plan and provides advice on how to follow it. This chapter also tells you all you need to know about when to eat and when to fast. Here, I also give you some details about the other versions of time-restricted intermittent fasts if you want to try a plan other than the 16:8.

Clarifying What Time-Restricted Intermittent Fasting Is

Most people eat from the time they wake up until the time they go to bed. When you practice time-restricted eating, you basically limit the number of hours you eat in a day. The popularity of this form of intermittent fasting lies in the fact that when you switch from the traditional style of eating (three meals and snacks) to time-restricted eating, you'll naturally eat less calories and lose weight — no counting calories, no restricting favorite foods — hence easier than old-fashioned dieting. Those people who are unsuccessful with this type of fasting are those individuals who allow themselves to cram all their typical calories into their eating window.

REMEMBER

Time-restricted intermittent fasting is a type of plan that limits your food intake to a certain number of hours each day — your eating window. You choose the most sustainable time frame and hours that work best for your lifestyle. This plan isn't a license to binge eat any and everything you want during your eating window. The goal for weight and fat loss is still to create a daily *calorie deficit* (you eat less calories on a daily basis than you used to).

Although the 16:8 is probably the most common and the easiest plan for you to start with, other intermittent plans, including the 17:7, 18:6, and 20:4 are options you can choose. Here I specifically discuss the 16:8 intermittent fasting plan, how it works, and see if this is the intermittent fast you want to start following today.

Trying the 16:8 time-restricted plan

The 16:8 intermittent fasting is quite effortless and the simplest plan for you to start with. With the 16:8 plan, you restrict eating to an 8-hour window such as 10 a.m. to 6 p.m. and fast 6 p.m. to 10 a.m. the following day. The 16:8 intermittent fast was first popularized by Martin Berkhan with his book *The Leangains Method.*

With the 16:8 time-restricted intermittent fasting plan, you choose the 8 hours when you eat all your calories and continue that pattern daily. The 8-hour eating window is the most lenient of all the intermittent fasts, because the 8-hour time frame gives you a wide eating latitude compared to other time-restricted eating patterns. Plus, you can easily map out the eating window hours in your day that most coincide with your work and social activities. You could start today and simply move breakfast to 10 a.m. and stop eating at 6 p.m. — whatever works for you!

TIP

If your goal is weight loss, you want to be sure that the number of hours you eat is less than what you typically allow yourself. In other words, if you're used to eating over a 10-hour period, you want to ensure that you reduce your eating window to much less (the lower, the better). If you have good results with the 16:8 or you're more ambitious, you can reduce your eating window, which can range from 4 to 12 hours a day, meaning 16- to 20-hour fasts.

Seeing why the 16:8 plan is easy

The 16:8 plan is popular because it's a more conservative time-restricted feeding protocol than all the other forms of intermittent fasting. In fact, this eating pattern is much more like a normal eating pattern than other intermittent fasting plans. Many people even adhere to this eating pattern unintentionally; it translates into a pattern of skipping breakfast and not eating after dinner each day. The 16:8 method is also popular for beginners because people typically sleep for about half of the 16 fasting hours.

TIP

To clarify, people lose weight following time-restricted intermittent fasts because by restricting eating windows to less than before, they automatically eat less calories on a daily basis. The concept is, if you restrict the amount of time you can spend eating, you'll eat less food than you used to. If you make up for the missed meals by overindulging during your eating windows, you will *not* lose weight.

Consider this example of a person following the 16:8 time-restricted intermittent fasting: John's goals are to stay healthy and fit and lose some body fat. Before John, 45, began intermittent fasting, he normally ate his first meal at 8 a.m. and kept eating (and drinking) until around 10 p.m. He therefore ate all his food in a 14-hour window each day. John decided to begin a time-restricted intermittent fast, so he reduced this eating window number (the number of hours he consumed food each day) to an 8-hour eating window. He found it easiest for him to only eat during a window of 8 hours (repeating the same 8-hour window day in and day out), which essentially removed two of his meals or snacks.

John revised his schedule by starting eating at noon and stopping eating at 8 p.m. — a time frame that worked best for his work and family schedules. Plus, he continued with his daily cardio workout first thing in the morning, practiced rhythmic relaxation breathing exercises for 5 minutes just before lunch, and squeezed a strength-training workout in — twice a week — just after work. John followed this plan for six months and lost 5 pounds of body fat plus reduced his fasting blood sugar level to less than 100 mg/dl, lowered his LDL cholesterol, and raised his HDL cholesterol numbers.

Losing the fat and keeping the muscle

The best way to lose the fat and not your muscle mass that you have worked so hard to gain is to continue your regular strength-training workouts during your time-restricted fasting plan. Chapter 14 gives you an in-depth discussion of which exercises are best and how often you should be performing them.

WARNING

Make sure to get consent from your personal physician before you engage in an exercise program, especially exercise combined with intermittent fasting.

If you're a fit and muscular person and are following a time-restricted intermittent fast to garner the health benefits, maintain your lean body mass, and lose some body fat, then I have some good news — some sound scientific data supports the effectiveness of this strategy.

A study out of Italy looked at the effect of putting resistance-trained, lifetime steroid-free athletes on an 8-week program of 16:8 time-restricted fasting.

Thirty-four muscular, fit men (average age 30 years old) were divided into two groups: the regular diet and the 16:8 diet. Both groups of men continued their regular weight-training routines. During the 8-week experimental period, the 16:8 subjects consumed 100 percent of their calories (daily calories calculated to maintain current body weight) divided into three meals consumed at 1 p.m., 4 p.m., and 8 p.m., and fasting for the remaining 16 hours per 24-hour period. The control group ingested their caloric intake (calculated to maintain current body weight) as three meals consumed at 8 a.m., 1 p.m., and 8 p.m.

The results? Both groups maintained their same level of muscle mass. However, only the 16:8 group showed significant health and body composition gains. The intermittent fasters lost a sizable amount of body fat (2½ pounds) and reduced their bodies' level of inflammation. Furthermore, only the intermittent fasting group showed a decrease in blood sugar and insulin levels. Importantly, the fasting group also demonstrated a significant increase in adiponectin levels.

TECHNICAL STUFF

Adiponectin is a hormone produced and secreted exclusively by *adipocytes* (fat cells). Adiponectin functions to regulate the metabolism of fats and blood sugar. In humans, blood levels of adiponectin are significantly lower in people with insulin-resistance and type 2 diabetes. The increase in adiponectin and decrease in insulin levels seen in the 16:8 intermittent fasting group is due to the ability of intermittent fasting to increase insulin sensitivity — a well-known effect of increased adiponectin levels. Moreover, adiponectin has an anti-inflammatory effect that led to the reduction of inflammatory markers seen in the fasting group.

A key point of the time-restricted fasting approach utilized in the study was that total daily calorie intake remained the same in both groups, with only the time between meals altered for the fasting group. The mere timing of food affected body composition and health markers. Time-restricted intermittent fasting with 16 hours of fasting and 8 hours of eating is a beneficial training strategy for resistance-trained athletes to improve health-related biomarkers, decrease fat mass, and at least maintain muscle mass. Bodybuilders could adopt this kind of regimen during their maintenance phases of training, commonly referred to as *cutting*, in which the goal is to maintain muscle mass while reducing fat mass.

Recognizing how much is too much

After you decide on a specific daily eating period, what and how often should you eat? That depends on your goals. If you're partaking in intermittent fasting to lose weight, then you must ensure that your eating period doesn't turn into an eat-everything food fest. For weight loss, the primary reason for its success is that intermittent fasting helps you eat fewer calories overall. If you binge and eat massive amounts during your eating windows, you probably won't lose any weight at all and may even gain some.

WARNING

A common initial side effect of starting an intermittent fasting program includes feeling hungry and irritable, also known as being *hangry.* You're probably familiar with the feeling; you're hungry and growing hungrier with every passing minute. Your hunger is making you increasingly unpleasant to be around, upset, irritable, angry. You are hangry!

Understand that you can control these feelings (flip to Chapter 15 for help). The good news is that they usually pass after two weeks to a month as your body and brain become accustomed to this new lifestyle. During your hours of fasting, try to consume plentiful amounts of noncaloric beverages, such as water, black coffee, and tea as well as eating nutritious foods during your eating windows. Doing so will take the edge off your appetite and help prevent you from becoming hangry.

Visualizing a Time-Restricted Fasting Plan — A Sample 1-Week Calendar

Choose the eating window that works best for your lifestyle, make your own calendar (see Figure 9-1), and start now to begin your life enhancing intermittent fasting journey. This less drastic type of time-restricted intermittent fasting may be a good choice for you as a newbie. It's fairly easy to follow and many people find it the most doable plan for their lifestyle.

Time/period	Sunday	Monday	Tuesday	Wednesday	Thursday	Friday	Saturday
Midnight							
4 a.m.							
8 a.m.							
12 p.m.							
2 p.m.			EATING WINDOW				
4 p.m.							
8 p.m.							
After 8 p.m.							

FIGURE 9-1:
A sample 1-week 16:8 intermittent fasting plan.

TIP

I suggest you start with 16:8 for the first few weeks. After you have some success, you may consider increasing your fasting window (go with 18 hours of fasting and 6 hours of eating). Regardless of the amount of time you choose for your eating window and your fasting window, remember to keep your fasting goal and feasting goals in mind (see Chapter 8).

Chapter **10**

Enlisting the Warrior Intermittent Fasting Plan

ear the word "warrior" and you may envision a Roman gladiator with his well-oiled and perfectly defined rippled muscles bulging from under his scant armor — a fearless warrior fighting lions by hand in the Colosseum. Don't misinterpret the use of the word to describe a style of intermittent fasting to mean that simply following this intermittent fast will turn you into a warrior.

That's not to say that you can't get leaner and bigger on this plan. This chapter examines the Warrior style of intermittent fasting and gives you just what you need to know. Read on to see if this intermittent fast best fits your lifestyle and goals.

Describing What The Warrior Intermittent Fasting Plan Is

Often referred to as the *20:4 intermittent fast*, the Warrior intermittent fasting plan is just another form of time-restricted fasting. Here, the window of eating is 4 hours a day, hence a much stricter version than other time-restricted intermittent fasts. The most popular time-restricted fast is the 16:8 version, where the eating window is a much broader time frame of 8 hours and is often recommended for beginner intermittent fasters. (Refer to Chapter 9 for more details about the 16:8 version.)

Twenty hours of fasting and a 4-hour eating window is spartan. During your eating window, you can eat more than one meal. The Warrior plan definitely isn't the easiest variation of intermittent fasting, and the plan doesn't have any modifications. If you deviate from the 20:4 protocol, you won't be following the Warrior intermittent fasting plan anymore.

WARNING

The Warrior intermittent fast means fasting for 20 hours overnight and during the day, and then eating during a 4-hour window in the evening. If your goal is weight loss, you need to ensure that you don't consume too many calories during your 4-hour feasting period or you'll gain weight. Despite the incredible freedom of being able to eat whatever you want, you should strive to make your food choices balanced and rich in nutrients — for the sake of your overall health. If you are curious how many calories you can squeeze into your 4 hours, flip to Chapter 3 and do the calorie calcs.

WHERE THE TRUE WARRIOR DIET FIRST STARTED AND WHAT'S WRONG WITH IT

Ori Hofmekler, a former member of the Israeli Special Forces, who eventually transitioned into the field of health and fitness, first popularized the Warrior Diet. In his bestseller, *The Warrior Diet,* first published in 2002, Hofmekler directs individuals to aim for literally "feasting" during the 4-hour window — encouraged to eat 80 to 90 percent of their daily calories during this time frame. He also allows small amounts of food or snacks (certain fruits, juices, veggies, eggs, and dairy) to be consumed during the 20-hour fast.

The Warrior Diet approach evolved into the One Meal a Day (OMAD) Diet. OMAD is quite simple: You eat one meal per day, consisting of whatever you want, typically at your regular dinnertime.

The Warrior Diet is basically an extremely long fast and a short feast. The Romans believed it was healthier to eat only one meal a day — hence the association between Roman gladiator warriors and this style of eating. The Romans believed that eating more than one meal was a form of gluttony.

An extreme variant of the Warrior intermittent fasting plan is the One Meal a Day (OMAD) plan where you eat only one meal a day of anything you want, usually at dinnertime. The difference between OMAD and a time-restricted intermittent fasting plan is instead of fasting for the typical window, like 16 hours (or 20 hours in the case of the Warrior plan), you fast for a whopping 23 hours (including the time you spend sleeping).

Eyeing the Pros and Cons to the Warrior Intermittent Fasting Plan

Table 10-1 identifies some of the main pros and cons to the Warrior intermittent plan:

TABLE 10-1　**Pros and Cons to the Eat-Stop-Eat Plan**

Pros	Cons
You may like the challenge. Sticking to the Warrior intermittent fast is a great way to practice discipline.	This plan may be difficult for the intermittent fasting beginner. It's challenging to go from 3 meals a day to fasting for 20 hours.
You may eat less. People who follow this plan tend to report filling up quickly and losing the desire to overeat. Less food means weight loss.	If you're an endurance athlete, the Warrior Diet isn't your best option. It's too difficult to consume the extraordinarily high-calorie requirements of these athletes in such a short eating window.
You may obsess about food less. People who follow this plan often report thinking less about food and not feeling deprived.	A full 20-hour fast, practiced daily, may negatively affect your social life.

WARNING

If you choose to follow the Warrior intermittent fasting plan, you *must* ensure that you're getting in all the nutrients your body needs during your 4-hour eating window. Flip to Part 5 and peruse the healthiest foods to eat and try some of the delicious and nutritious recipes.

Exercising during Your Warrior Intermittent Fast

Yes, you can and should exercise during your Warrior intermittent fast. Ideally, if your goal is to add muscle and shed body fat, you must incorporate weight training into your exercise plan. Make sure your resistance exercise bouts are during your eating window whereas your cardio should take place during your fast. Refer to Chapter 14 for an in-depth discussion of exercise recommendations and timing.

WARNING

Make sure to get consent from your personal physician before you engage in an exercise program, especially exercise combined with intermittent fasting.

EXPLORING WHAT THE REAL WARRIORS ATE

The buzz around the training room lately is the controversial 2018 Netflix documentary *The Game Changers* about plant-based eating, protein, and strength. The movie has both broadened the appeal of plant-based diets and drawn massive criticism. Executive produced by James Cameron, Arnold Schwarzenegger, and Jackie Chan, the documentary follows James Wilks, an elite Special Forces trainer and winner of The Ultimate Fighter, who after an injury researches and applies a plant-based eating strategy. Low and behold, his athletic performance peaks, which he attributes to his new diet.

The documentary mixes groundbreaking science with anecdotal stories of struggle and triumph from Wilks. The film features some of the strongest, fastest, and toughest athletes on the planet. Wilks' journey exposes outdated myths about food (plant protein versus animal protein) that not only affect human performance, but also the health of the planet. The film highlights the recent study analyzing the ancient bones of gladiators excavated from the graves of 22 gladiators from about 1,800 years ago, buried in the Roman town of Ephesus (now Turkey). The bones revealed these men ate diets of mostly wheat, barley, and beans, hence the moniker Barley Men.

Furthermore, Roman texts from 2,000 years ago show that gladiators ate a specific diet termed *gladiatoriam saginam*, meaning a diet based primarily on wheat, barley, and beans. Contemporary accounts of gladiator life also refer derogatorily to the warriors as *hordearii* — literally *barley men*. The word *hordearii* relates to the fact that gladiators were probably given grain of an inferior quality. Roman gladiators were mainly recruited from among prisoners of war, slaves, and condemned offenders, hence the lower grade nutrition.

Visualizing a Warrior Intermittent Fast — A Sample 1-Week Calendar

Are you considering starting a Warrior intermittent fast? Figure 10-1 is an example of a one-week Warrior intermittent fast, also referred to as a 20:4 style, to give you a better idea of how you can choose to space out your eating schedule.

Time/period	Sunday	Monday	Tuesday	Wednesday	Thursday	Friday	Saturday
8 a.m.	Fast	Fast	Fast	Fast	Fast	Fast	Fast
12 p.m.							
2 p.m.							
4 p.m.							
4 p.m.–8 p.m.	EAT						
After 8 p.m.	Fast	Fast	Fast	Fast	Fast	Fast	Fast
Midnight							
2 a.m.							

© John Wiley & Sons, Inc.

FIGURE 10-1: A sample 1-week Warrior intermittent fasting plan.

The Warrior intermittent fasting plan is no walk in the park, but it can be an extremely effective way to reach your health goals, if done properly. Just be sure to eat whole, nutritious foods during your eating window.

REMEMBER

A plant-based whole foods diet such as the Mediterranean Diet is the best diet to combine with your intermittent fasting lifestyle for promoting better health and longevity. Eat like a gladiator and follow a plant-based diet.

The key is choosing a style of intermittent fasting that works for you over the long term. If you want to try intermittent fasting, the Warrior intermittent fasting plan probably isn't the best place to start. You may want to begin with the 16:8 intermittent fasting protocol that I discuss in Chapter 9 or the 5:2 method that I explain in Chapter 12 because the Warrior intermittent fast is tough to stick to, especially for beginners.

Chapter **11**

Attempting the Alternate Day Intermittent Fasting Plan

ntermittent fasting has a variety of schedules for you to choose from. Some are much more difficult to follow than others, however, investigating them all can help you choose the plan that's right for your personal lifestyle.

Another option, the Alternate Day intermittent fasting, also referred to as the *4:3 plan*, has the most scientific data supporting its efficacy and safety of all the plans. Read on and see if perhaps the Alternate Day intermittent fasting plan is right for you.

Explaining the Different Versions of Alternate Day Intermittent Fasting Plans

Strict Alternate Day intermittent fasting is one of the most extreme dietary interventions because you avoid all food for 36-hour periods. One day you eat, the next day you don't, repeat. In other words, you fast on one day and then eat what you want the next day, then fast the next day, and so on. In other words, you eat 4 days during the week and fast 3 nonconsecutive days.

Alternate Day intermittent fasting schedules aren't all the same. The following list mentions some of the different ways that Alternate Day intermittent fasting plans can occur:

>> You switch back and forth between days when you eat more and days when you eat less.

>> You eat nothing or next to nothing on your fast days and as much as you want on your feast days.

>> You cut your usual food intake by a third to a half on your fasting days and allow yourself to eat more than your usual food intake on your feasting days. This is sometimes called *calorie cycling*.

>> You do a complete fast on Monday, Wednesdays, and Fridays, so your intermittent fast is a three-day endeavor. This version is popular because you have the weekends to enjoy eating with friends and family.

Even though some Alternate Day fasting schedules only allow calorie-free drinks on fasting days, others allow small amounts of food (typically a maximum of 25 percent of your total daily calories) on fasting days.

Understanding the Science of the Alternate Day Intermittent Fasting Plan

As a scientist, the Alternate Day intermittent fasting plan is one of my favorites because I like to see the data. Low and behold, there is myriad sound scientific research regarding Alternate Day fasting and the associated miraculous health benefits.

For example, the journal *Cell Metabolism* published the results of a randomized clinical trial (the gold standard of scientific studies showing cause and effect) that examined the effects on the body of Alternate Day intermittent fasting. The largest study of its kind to look at the effects of strict Alternate Day intermittent fasting in healthy people showed a wide range of health benefits. The participants alternated 36 hours of zero-calorie intake with 12 hours of unlimited eating.

In this study, Austrian researchers enrolled 60 participants (subjects in both groups were all of normal weight and were healthy, aged 35 to 65 years old) into a four-week study and randomized the subjects into either an Alternate Day fasting group or a control group, the latter of which could eat as much as the group wanted. Here are the results detected in the intermittent fasting group:

>> The group had evidence of a continuous amount of ketones in the blood, even on nonfasting days. The ketone overflow has been shown to promote health in various ways (see Chapter 5 for a more in-depth discussion of the wonders of ketones).

>> The group had reduced levels of a blood marker linked to age-associated disease and inflammation called *soluble intercellular adhesion molecule-1*.

>> The group had lowered levels of a thyroid hormone called *triiodothyronine* without impaired thyroid gland function. Low levels of this hormone have been linked to longevity in humans.

>> The group had lowered levels of LDL cholesterol and triglycerides.

>> The group lost weight and body fat (a 9 percent loss of body fat, especially a reduction of harmful belly fat).

These intermittent fasters drank only water on their fasting days and continued to participate in their usual activity level. Figure 11-1 depicts the intermittent fasting schedule used in this study (the circle-backslash symbol indicates complete water-only fasting).

FIGURE 11-1:
Alternate Day intermittent fasting pattern used in this study.

Monday	Tuesday	Wednesday	Thursday	Friday	Saturday	Sunday
🚫	Feast	🚫	Feast	🚫	Feast	🚫
Feast	🚫	Feast	🚫	Feast	🚫	Feast

© John Wiley & Sons, Inc.

WARNING

The subjects in this study were healthy, young and middle-aged, active adults. If you have any medical issues or conditions, you must get your physician's consent before embarking on any intermittent fast. Flip to Chapter 7 for guidance on who should and shouldn't begin a program of intermittent fasting.

Additional research on the Alternate Day intermittent fasting plan has shown a reduction in the following:

>> Asthma

>> Heart arrhythmias

>> Insulin resistance

>> Menopausal hot flashes

>> Seasonal allergies

Benefiting from the Alternate Day Intermittent Fasting Plan

Another study examined the Alternate Day intermittent fasting plan and highlighted several benefits. Dr. Krista Varady, an associate professor of nutrition at the University of Illinois, refers to the Alternate Day intermittent fasting plan as the *Every Other Day Diet*, also referred to as the *Up-Day, Down-Day* plan. She has published a book and numerous well-constructed studies. This plan involves a fast day where individuals consume 25 percent of their calorie needs, alternated with a feed day where people eat as much as they want.

In a 12-week randomized clinical trial published in the *Nutrition Journal*, Varady recruited both normal weight and overweight subjects. After 12 weeks on the Alternate Day intermittent fast, the health benefits were compelling. The subjects

>> **Lost weight.** Body weight was reduced by 6 percent (11 pounds) by the end of the trial.

>> **Lowered body fat.** Body fat decreased by 7.7 pounds with no change in muscle mass.

>> **Felt full.** Dietary satisfaction and feelings of fullness increased from baseline to post-treatment.

>> **Showed positive changes in markers of heart disease risk.** A significant reduction in triglyceride concentration (20 percent) was noted after 12 weeks. Plus, LDL particle size also increased post-treatment (LDL is bad cholesterol and bigger is healthier).

>> **Experienced lower inflammation.** Decreases in circulating c-reactive protein (CRP) concentrations were observed. *CRP* is a protein made by the liver that is a marker of inflammation in the body.

>> **Had increased insulin sensitivity.** An increase in *adiponectin,* the protein hormone that exhibits anti-diabetic, anti-inflammatory, and anti-atherogenic effects, and a hormone that functions as an insulin sensitizer.

Alternate Day intermittent fasting has had numerous additional scientific research findings as to its benefits. These include the following:

>> **Increased weight and fat loss.** A 2013 study published in the *Nutrition Journal* found that following this intermittent fast for 12 weeks caused a loss of nearly 8 pounds of body fat. If middle-aged spread is a problem, another recent study noted that people aged 50 to 59 years achieved greater weight loss with Alternate Day intermittent fasting compared to people of other age groups.

>> **Improved heart health.** Heart disease is the leading cause of death globally. Alternate Day intermittent fasting helps reduce the risk of heart disease in many ways that would be more fruitful when combined with a healthy Mediterranean lifestyle, which is proven to promote heart health. (Refer to Chapter 17 for more about how a plant-based Mediterranean Diet can help you improve your heart health among other benefits.)

>> **Improved insulin sensitivity and blood sugar level.** High blood sugar levels occur when the body fails to produce enough insulin or can't properly use available insulin (referred to as *insulin resistance*). Persistently high sugar levels can lead to diabetes. Studies have shown that Alternate Day intermittent fasting can help reduce fasting blood sugar levels by reducing the blood levels of insulin and increasing insulin sensitivity.

>> **Promoted autophagy.** *Autophagy* is the process that recycles unused, damaged, and potentially harmful cell components. Refer to Chapter 6 for more information about autophagy.

>> **Promoted longevity (in animals).** Restricting total calorie intake, which can be achieved from Alternate Day intermittent fasting, has been shown to significantly prolong the lifespan in animal studies. Refer to Chapter 5 for more information on calorie restriction (CR) research.

Exercising during Your Alternate Day Intermittent Fast

You can and should exercise during your Alternate Day intermittent fasting program. You may want to consider when and how to schedule in your different types of exercise bouts during your Alternate Day intermittent fasting calendar. Refer to Chapter 14 for an in-depth discussion of exercise recommendations and timing.

You may wonder why you'd want to add exercise to your Alternate Day intermittent fasting regimen. The answer is simple — so you can supercharge your weight loss! The journal *Obesity* published a study that showed participants doubled their weight loss with cardio. Sixty overweight subjects were divided into four groups:

>> Alternate Day fasting alone (diet)

>> Diet plus cardio exercise

>> No diet or exercise

>> Exercise alone

The participants who combined the Alternate Day intermittent fasting plan with cardio exercise burned at least twice as much fat as each individual approach. The researchers also showed that the combination produced superior changes in body composition (a significant loss of body fat and retention of muscle mass) and reduced indicators of heart disease risk compared to individual treatments.

WARNING

Make sure to get consent from your personal physician before you engage in an exercise program, especially exercise combined with intermittent fasting.

Eyeing an Alternate Day Intermittent Fast — A Sample 1-Week Calendar

You may have seen a few different examples of Alternate Day intermittent fasting floating around the Internet. Figure 11-2 shows you an example of incorporating this plan into your life.

REMEMBER

Alternate Day fasting is another difficult form of intermittent fasting not recommended for beginners. You can choose to make it easier by allowing yourself the 25 percent of your typical calories on your fasting days. You'll still reap the massive health benefits regardless of which style you choose.

Sunday	Monday	Tuesday	Wednesday	Thursday	Friday	Saturday
Normal Eating	**FASTING**	Normal Eating	**FASTING**	Normal Eating	**FASTING**	Normal Eating

FIGURE 11-2:
A sample 1-week Alternate Day intermittent fasting plan.

© John Wiley & Sons, Inc.

Chapter **12**

Applying the 5:2 Intermittent Fasting Plan

The 5:2 intermittent fasting plan, also known as *The Fast Diet*, is one of the most well-liked forms of intermittent fasting. Perhaps it's even the most famous of the intermittent fasting regimens. Read on to see if this intermittent fast is best tailored to your personality type and needs.

Shedding Light on the 5:2 Intermittent Fasting Plan

The 5:2 intermittent fasting plan involves eating how you normally would on five days of the week and eating only 500 to 600 calories on the other two days. For one to two nonconsecutive days per week, you consume just water plus 500 calories (if you're a woman) or 600 calories (if you're a man) either in one meal or spread out over the day; your calorie intake should be a quarter of your daily needs. The other five or six days a week, you can eat whatever you want, whenever you want (you don't have to even think about restricting calories). You can choose whichever two days of the week you prefer, as long as you have at least one non-fasting day in between them.

For some people, this plan may be easier to follow than say the Alternate Day intermittent fast (that I discuss in Chapter 11). Only having to restrict food intake one or two days a week and then not having to worry about what to eat the other five to six days can be appealing to a large swath of people.

TECHNICAL STUFF

British broadcaster Michael Mosley popularized the 5:2 intermittent fasting plan. He purportedly came up with the 5:2 intermittent fast because he had been diagnosed with type 2 diabetes and wanted to reverse it without medication. In 2012, Mosley filmed the wildly popular BBC documentary *Michael Mosley Presents Horizon: Eat, Fast, and Live Longer.* He later published *The Fast Diet* in 2013.

Examining the Science of the 5:2 Intermittent Fasting Plan

The 5:2 intermittent fasting plan also has a large amount of scientific backing, and it's one of my favorites. Johns Hopkins neuroscientist Mark Mattson, PhD, has studied intermittent fasting and its underlying mechanisms for 25 years. He has published several controlled human studies that investigate the impacts of various intermittent fasting interventions, most often the 5:2 intermittent fasting plan.

His research demonstrated the following:

>> One hundred overweight women showed that those on the 5:2 intermittent fasting diet lost the same amount of weight as women who restricted calories, but they did better on measures of insulin sensitivity and reduced belly fat than those in the calorie-reduction group.

>> Two hundred twenty healthy, nonobese adults who practiced 5:2 intermittent fasting for two years showed signs of improved memory in a battery of cognitive tests. These results suggest that intermittent fasting may offer interventions that can stave off neurodegeneration and dementia.

It can take time for your body to adjust to intermittent fasting. For some, hunger pangs and irritability are common initial intermittent fasting side effects. The good news is, they tend to dissipate after two weeks to a month, as the body and brain become accustomed to the new eating regime.

According to the Johns Hopkins University website (www.hopkinsmedicine.org), which summarizes an article in *The New England Journal of Medicine,* here are what doctors believe 5:2 intermittent fasting can improve:

» **Cardiovascular health:** Studies support numerous heart health benefits of intermittent fasting including reduced blood pressure and resting heart rate as well as other heart-related measurements.

» **Brain performance:** Studies support improved cognitive ability with intermittent fasting. Studies discovered that intermittent fasting boosts verbal memory in adult humans.

» **Athletic performance and body composition:** One study shows significant fat loss while maintaining muscle mass in athletic men.

» **Blood sugar level:** Numerous studies have shown significant weight loss with intermittent fasting and normalization of blood glucose.

» **Wound healing:** Studies show intermittent fasting reduces tissue damage in surgery and improves surgical outcomes.

The 5:2 plan is another method of helping your body achieve autophagy, the state of cellular rejuvenation. For more information on the joys of autophagy, refer to Chapter 6.

Exercising during Your 5:2 Intermittent Fast

Exercise is a perfect addition to any intermittent fast, including the 5:2 intermittent fast. Doing your cardio during the fasted state is highly beneficial because you get an additive effect of increased insulin sensitivity and fat loss — a golden combination. Refer to Chapter 14 for an in-depth discussion of exercise recommendations and timing.

WARNING

Make sure to get consent from your personal physician before you engage in an exercise program, especially exercise combined with intermittent fasting.

Visualizing a 5:2 Intermittent Fast — A Sample 1-Week Calendar

The 5:2 approach to intermittent fasting is quite simple. If you're a woman, consume a maximum of 500 calories on your fasting days, 600 calories if you're a man. Figure 12-1 shows an example calendar you can follow with the 5:2 intermittent fast. If you're trying this plan, flip to Chapter 22 for some delicious and nutritious calorie-controlled plant-based recipes that adhere to the calorie limitations.

The popular 5:2 intermittent fast may just be the right choice for you. Remember to eat healthfully during your eating days and stick to the calorie level that fits your gender on your fasting days. Also, give the plan time to work and rest assured, you'll soon begin to watch the magic happen.

Sunday	Monday	Tuesday	Wednesday	Thursday	Friday	Saturday
Normal Eating	Restricted Calories Women: 500 calories Men: 600 calories	Normal Eating	Normal Eating	Restricted Calories Women: 500 calories Men: 600 calories	Normal Eating	Normal Eating

FIGURE 12-1:
A sample 1-week 5:2 intermittent fasting plan.

© *John Wiley & Sons, Inc.*

Chapter **13**

Starting the Eat-Stop-Eat Intermittent Fasting Plan

You can implement an intermittent fasting protocol into your routine in many ways, and one method that's becoming increasingly popular is known as the *Eat-Stop-Eat* intermittent fast. This chapter reviews everything you need to know about this kind of plan, including how to implement it, whether it's effective for weight loss, and any possible drawbacks you need to consider before diving in.

Perusing the Eat-Stop-Eat Intermittent Fasting Plan

In following the Eat-Stop-Eat intermittent fasting program, also referred to as the *24-hour fast,* you choose one or two nonconsecutive days per week during which you completely abstain from eating — or fast — for a full 24-hour period. During the 24-hour fast you can't consume any food except for calorie-free drinks. So, in effect, you're aiming for a complete break from food for 24 hours at a time.

Though doing so may seem counterintuitive, you can still eat something on each calendar day of the week. For example, you may eat normally until 6 p.m. on a Tuesday, and then fast until 6 p.m. on Wednesday, resuming regular eating at that time. According to Brad Pilon, the Canadian author who popularized this intermittent fasting plan in his book, *Eat Stop Eat,* if you can't make it the full 24 hours, 20 hours will also work (albeit then it technically would be the 20:4 plan, also called the Warrior plan; see Chapter 10). *Translation:* You can eat whatever you want 5 or 6 days a week.

REMEMBER

If you're only fasting once a week, this plan is ideal for keeping up or starting a daily exercise routine. Just make sure you get your physician's consent before starting any exercise routine.

The next sections discuss the pros and cons to the Eat–Stop–Eat plan and examine some of research to show its benefit.

Examining the pros and cons

Similar to the 5:2 plan that I discuss in Chapter 12, the Eat–Stop–Eat intermittent fast has pros and cons to following it. Table 13-1 lists some of the pros and cons:

TABLE 13-1   **Pros and Cons to the Eat-Stop-Eat Plan**

Pros	Cons
It's flexible and easier to follow compared to other more stringent fasting programs because you only fast for 24 hours at a time.	Refraining from food for entire 24 hours can be difficult.
Works well for people who have certain days of the week where they're either particularly busy or social and other days where they're less social where fasting would be easier.	There's a danger of overeating after the eating period begins.
Myriad health benefits, including weight loss, increased fat burning, maintenance of muscle mass, reduction in hunger hormones, and increased insulin sensitivity.	Fasting 24 hours once or twice a week may not be sustainable over the long term.
Doesn't have food limits or any other restrictions.	Potential for negative side effects (see Chapter 15).
Doesn't promote calorie counting or food weighing.	Hard to participate in social interactions that involve food, such as parties or dinners out with friends.

TIP

Keep in mind, my recommendations for obtaining the results you want are as follows, regardless of the intermittent fasting plan you choose:

>> Practice consistency.

>> Eat mindful.

>> Consume a plant-based whole foods, Mediterranean-style nutritious diet when feasting.

>> Don't treat your nonfasting days as a food-fest free for all.

Seeing what the research says

A lot of scientific research has been centered on the 5:2 diet, Alternate Day fasting, and the 16:8 versions of intermittent fasting. Although not referred to in the scientific literature as "Eat-Stop-Eat," there is a substantial amount of research on what's termed *weekly one-day fasting* or *periodic 24-hour fasting*, which is essentially the same plan as the Eat-Stop-Eat version of intermittent fasting.

Scientists at the Intermountain Medical Center in Salt Lake City, Utah, investigated the non-weight loss health effects of a 24-hour water-only fast. The goal of the research was to understand the physiological changes that occur in the body during a 24-hour fasting episode. Referred to as the FEELGOOD clinical trial, it was conducted over a two-day participation period and consisted of 30 healthy participants, randomized to either the fasting or the eating groups. Multiple indicators of health were collected and analyzed in both groups. Here are the findings exhibited in the fasting group:

>> **Human growth hormone:** Human growth hormone (HGH), which is secreted from the pituitary gland in the brain, was dramatically elevated during fasting. HGH builds muscle mass, boosts metabolism, and helps the body burn fat.

>> **Red blood cells:** Red blood cell count and hemoglobin were increased during fasting. During fasting cycles, the body promotes regeneration of the entire circulatory system, which benefits the cardiovascular health.

>> **Cholesterol and triglycerides:** Total cholesterol and high-density lipoprotein cholesterol increased, and triglycerides decreased during fasting. An increase in good HDL cholesterol and a reduction of bad fats, namely triglycerides, is highly protective against heart and vascular disease.

>> **Trimethylamine N-oxide:** Fasting significantly lowers blood levels of a compound called *trimethylamine N-oxide (TMAO)*. TMAO is a known biomarker of cardiovascular disease in humans that arises from intestinal microbiota.

(The gut microbiome are the trillions of microbes that reside in the intestinal tract.) People eat food, and the gut bacteria break it down and produce a compound called trimethylamine (TMA). The liver then converts TMA into the compound, TMAO. The trouble with TMAO is that data show high levels contribute to a heightened risk for clot-related events such as heart attack and stroke. Furthermore, scientists have proven that high blood levels of TMAO are associated with higher rates of premature death. Periodic fasting, therefore, beneficially alters the microbiome, away from the pro-cardiovascular disease composition.

>> **Amino acids:** Fasting significantly reduced blood levels of the amino acids proline and tyrosine. Lower circulating proline and tyrosine are linked with less insulin resistance, better cognitive function, and less depression.

>> **Urea:** The fasting group exhibited a significantly reduced blood urea level. *Urea* is a nitrogen-containing breakdown product of protein metabolism that is excreted in the urine. A reduced blood level of urea can reduce blood pressure in people with high blood pressure.

Visualizing an Eat-Stop-Eat Intermittent Fast— A Sample 1-Week Calendar

Thinking the Eat–Stop–Eat plan is the style of intermittent fasting you want to embark on? Figure 13-1 shows an example of a single day Eat–Stop–Eat intermittent fast, which may be a method you might want to consider if you're a beginner.

FIGURE 13-1:
A sample 1-week Eat-Stop-Eat intermittent fasting plan.

Sunday	Monday	Tuesday	Wednesday	Thursday	Friday	Saturday
Normal Eating	**FASTING**	Normal Eating	Normal Eating	Normal Eating	Normal Eating	Normal Eating

© John Wiley & Sons, Inc.

You are in charge, you make the calls, and you design the program that works best for you. Follow this suggested eating regimen for the best of both worlds and get ready to enjoy this remarkable health and wellness journey. And don't forget to include exercise, like I discuss in Chapter 14, with your plan under your doctor's supervision.

4

Customizing Your Complete Intermittent Fasting Plan

Optimize your intermittent fast of choice with your secret weapon: your daily exercise routine — proven to enhance your results, improve your health and fitness, and keep you motivated and focused.

Consider the possible struggles and challenges you may face during your intermittent fasting journey and how to overcome any potential obstacles.

Explore your connection with food and decide for yourself if you need to create a healthier relationship.

IN THIS CHAPTER

» **Understanding the importance of exercise**

» **Creating your daily exercise routine**

» **Exploring the benefits of the different types of exercise**

Chapter **14**

Combining Daily Exercise with Your Intermittent Fasting Plan

Expanding abdominal girth and shrinking muscle mass are too often the unfortunate side effects of aging for most Americans. The most effective way to tame and even prevent these phenomena is to partake in a regular exercise program. Combining a daily exercise routine with a program of intermittent fasting is the ultimate metabolism booster that will have a profound positive effect on your body and your health.

WARNING

Although exercising and intermittent fasting is perfectly safe for most people, others may not feel comfortable doing any form of exercise while fasting. If you haven't been exercising regularly, now isn't the time to begin an intensive workout program. Always get the permission from your doctor or healthcare provider before starting any exercise program, especially if combining exercise with a program of intermittent fasting.

This chapter focuses on the different types of exercise and how to safely incorporate them into your life with your intermittent fasting regimen. You may have several different questions like what type of exercise should accompany your plan, whether you should exercise during the fed or fasted state, and can you practice intermittent fasting and still build muscle. I answer all these questions and more here. Most importantly, you *can* safely exercise during your intermittent fasting regimen, with several caveats.

Capturing What You Need to Know about Intermittent Fasting and Exercise

Regular exercise can promote health in similar ways to intermittent fasting. Combining the two lifestyles is a powerful strategy to do the following:

>> **Promote greater weight and fat loss.** Exercise burns calories by contributing to your total daily metabolic burn. This calorie burn helps you lose weight faster by creating a greater *calorie deficit* (you burn more calories than you consume). When you combine intermittent fasting with daily exercise, you rev your metabolism to the max, which inevitably speeds weight and fat loss. Cardio exercise has also been proven to target belly fat. Combine daily cardio with your intermittent fasting plan of choice and you have a potent treatment for whittling away that stubborn belly fat once and for all.

>> **Provide additional psychological benefits.** Regular exercise can have a profoundly positive impact on mental health, proven to prevent and treat depression, anxiety, and more. Cardio exercise elevates your mood by promoting the release of *endorphins,* which are feel-good chemicals released by your brain. A regular exercise program also relieves stress, improves memory, and enhances quality of sleep.

>> **Further reduce insulin resistance.** Exercising regularly can increase insulin sensitivity and stimulate the muscle's uptake of blood sugar. In fact, just a single bout of moderate intensity exercise can increase blood sugar uptake by at least 40 percent! Combine daily exercise with intermittent fasting — also known to reduce insulin resistance — and you have a one-two punch to protect against type 2 diabetes.

>> **Further reduce inflammation.** Exercise reduces markers of inflammation (as does intermittent fasting) — inflammation is a key driver of many chronic diseases. Body fat mass and fat cell tissue release harmful inflammatory chemicals. Therefore, reducing body fat automatically lowers inflammation. Regardless of if you lose weight, the act of exercise heightens muscle production of natural anti-inflammatory substances.

>> **Double up on protecting your heart.** Regular exercise reduces bad LDL cholesterol, blood triglycerides, inflammatory markers, blood sugar, and insulin resistance — all risk factors for heart disease. Exercise also increases your levels of HDL cholesterol, the good cholesterol that lowers heart disease risk, by flushing artery-clogging LDL cholesterol out of your system.

>> **Provide additional cancer prevention benefits.** Exercise can help you lower your risk of many types of cancer including breast, colorectal, and uterine cancers. Exercise speeds digestion, which may reduce the time that potentially harmful substances are in contact with the colon.

>> **Help promote a healthier brain.** Exercise improves blood flow and memory, and it stimulates chemical changes in the brain that enhance learning, mood, and thinking. The same endorphins released during exercise that make you feel better also help you concentrate and increase mentally acuity for performing tasks at hand.

>> **Help fight age-related decline.** Daily exercise has been linked to a longer life. In fact, Harvard University researchers recently noted that as little as 15 minutes of physical activity a day can boost your life span by three years. Regarding aging, exercise stimulates the growth of new brain cells that help prevent age-related decline.

TIP

Exercise is the ultimate free fountain of youth. Drink from it daily and reap the benefits this "medicine" will provide you. It helps you lose body fat, fight disease, stay mentally fit, and increase longevity. The only side effect is euphoria.

You ideally should incorporate three different types of exercise into your life as an accompaniment to your intermittent fasting program. They are

>> Cardio (fitness slang for *cardiovascular* or *aerobic conditioning*)

>> Strength training

>> Mind-body exercises

Figure 14-1 depicts the recommended daily frequency of partaking in each form of exercise.

REMEMBER

Health authorities all agree that Americans should partake in a *daily* exercise routine for better health. According to the CDC, adults should aim for at least 150 minutes a week of moderate intensity activity such as brisk walking and at least two days a week of activities that strengthen muscles.

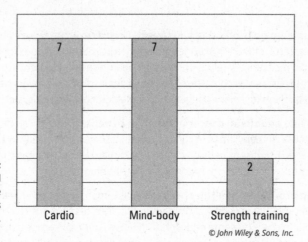

FIGURE 14-1: Recommended exercise frequency (days per week).

Transforming Your Body with Cardiovascular Conditioning

Aerobic exercise (*aerobic* means *with oxygen*) activities are also called cardio. *Cardiovascular exercise* is any activity, performed for an extended period of time, that increases heart rate and breathing while using the large muscle groups repetitively and rhythmically. During aerobic activity, you repeatedly move the large muscles in your arms, legs, and hips such as during jogging. Your heart rate increases, and you breathe faster and more deeply. This form of exercise maximizes the amount of oxygen in your blood and ultimately helps you use oxygen more efficiently.

Cardio or "heart" and *vascular* or "blood vessels" are descriptive words that provide a clue as to why this type of exercise is so important. Cardio exercise training progressively improves both the functioning and efficiency of your heart, lungs, and circulatory system.

These sections take a closer look at what kind of cardio you can do as well as when it's best to perform your exercise in combination with your intermittent fast.

Recognizing common cardio

To maintain health, the American College of Sports Medicine recommends performing a minimum of 30 minutes of moderate-intensity cardio activity on most, if not all, days of the week. Here is a list of common aerobic exercise activities:

>> Brisk walking

>> Cross-country skiing

>> Cycling

>> Hiking

>> Kickboxing

>> Rowing

>> Running

>> Swimming

In the gym, cardio machines include the treadmill, elliptical trainer, stationary cycle, stepping machine, rowing machine, aerobics classes, dancing, and spinning. But you don't need to go to a gym to do cardio.

TIP

If you're just getting started, walking is an ideal cardio choice. Don't underrate the benefits or difficulty of establishing a brisk walking program. Walking lets you choose the intensity level that works for you and results in fewer injuries than many other options. Walking doesn't require special equipment, and you can do it just about anywhere. Make sure that you purchase a great pair of walking shoes, stay hydrated, and dress for the elements.

Mapping out when and how

Your biggest question probably is when you should perform your cardio — during your fasted or fed state. The answer is to aim for engaging in physical activity while you're in your fasting state — creating a profound physiological impact on your body. Here is what happens during fasted cardio exercise:

>> **It improves insulin sensitivity more than intermittent fasting alone.** A program of regular cardio exercise sensitizes the muscles to insulin, because active muscles work like a vacuum, sucking up blood sugar. Scientific research shows that fasted cardio exercise has a compounded effect on making your body more sensitive to insulin — which means less weight gain/easier weight loss, better glucose control for those who are diabetic, pre-diabetic, or insulin-resistant, and more balanced blood sugar levels overall. Refer to Chapter 6 for more about the role of insulin in the body.

>> **It improves fat burning and revs up metabolic rate more than intermittent fasting alone.** Performing cardio will add to your metabolic burn as well as force your metabolism to use stored body fat for fuel as your carbohydrate

tank is already on empty. Therefore, timing your workout while you're fasting rather than feasting will get you better results.

>> **Human growth hormone production increases even more than with intermittent fasting alone.** Combining cardio during the fasted state results in an exponential stimulus to production of human growth hormone. According to the research, exercising while in a fasted state can dramatically increase human growth hormone release over and above the increase observed with fasting alone. For more information on the role growth hormone plays in muscle building, flip to Chapter 5.

Paying attention to your body

The most important advice to heed when exercising during your intermittent fasting is to listen to your body. Exercising during the fasting state heightens your risk of side effects. Stop exercising immediately and seek emergency care if you feel:

>> Chest pain or pressure

>> Extreme nausea

>> An irregular heartbeat

>> Pain in your neck, arm, jaw, shoulder, or other symptoms that cause concern of a heart attack

>> Unusual shortness of breath

>> Weak or dizzy

If you start to feel weak or dizzy, you may be experiencing low blood sugar or are dehydrated. If this happens, stop exercising and drink orange juice and eat a light meal. Always ensure you're hydrated and dress for the elements. If you're in pain, don't ignore it. Ignoring pain can lead to injury.

Note that both the intermittent fasting program you follow and your initial level of cardiovascular fitness will determine how you feel during your exercise bouts. If you're physically fit and used to aerobic exercise, you may initially encounter bouts of low blood sugar if you're exercising during your fasted state — it can lead to increased heart rate and poor athletic performance. These side effects will improve with continued exercise training as your body learns to rely more on ketones instead of blood sugar for fuel.

TIP

When designing your cardio program to go with your intermittent fasting plan, keep the intensity and duration of your cardio sessions lower than previously practiced. A progressive increase in intensity and duration will allow your body to adapt to this combination without potential side effects. Do load up on nutrient-dense good carbs, lean protein, and healthy fats during your feeding periods to give you the energy for your exercise bouts and to ensure that your workouts are effective in helping you achieve your goals while following your intermittent fasting plan. Always remember to stay hydrated before, during, and after your exercise bouts.

Healing Your Body with Strength Training

You know regular exercise is one of the best actions you can take for better health. Unfortunately, many Americans ignore the one type of exercise that is essential for maintaining muscle and bone mass — strength training (also known as *resistance exercise*). In fact, only 6 percent of Americans practice muscle strengthening exercise the government recommended minimum of twice per week.

TIP

Just two sessions a week (full-body exercises, up to three sets of each exercise, 8 to 12 reps on each set) is all you need to begin to reap the myriad health benefits of resistance exercise. No gym required; a simple resistance band will do the trick.

If exercise is medicine, then strength training is like aspirin, the original wonder drug. Here I examine some of the miraculous health benefits you can derive from simply lifting some weights a couple times a week.

Slowing down aging

Strength training can do wonders in helping slow down the aging process. When people age, they lose muscle, which in turn, lowers metabolic rate and bone density. Scientists estimate that muscle starts to deteriorate beginning at age 30. After age 40, it's downhill with an average of 8 percent of muscle mass lost every decade. This phenomenon continues to accelerate at an even faster rate after age 60. Combine this with the fact that the average person gains about a pound of body fat a year starting in middle age, and you have aging bodies that undergo a striking change in composition. This reshaping of the body reduces your metabolic rate because muscle is more metabolically active than fat.

Loss of muscle also affects your bone density, increasing your risk of osteoporosis. The bones and muscles in your body work together in tandem, and they either become stronger together or weaker together. By stressing your bones, strength training can increase bone density and reduce the risk of osteoporosis. Whenever you lose muscle, you automatically lose bone — they go hand in hand. Studies show that age-related loss of muscle hastens the onset of diseases, limits mobility, reduces ability to perform activities of daily living, and is linked to premature death.

It's never too late to benefit from strength training. Studies have shown that combining intermittent fasting with a regular muscle strength training exercise routine can produce greater weight and fat loss results than fasting alone. This type of exercise can also prevent the loss of muscle and reduction in metabolism typically seen with traditional diets. Research continually confirms that the best way to burn fat and hold onto muscle is to combine a healthy moderately reduced calorie diet with strength training.

Building muscle: No magic, just hard work

Strength training — any type of workout that builds strength and muscle — is the *only way* you can prevent muscle loss and add to your lean body mass. Building muscle has extraordinary health benefits. It does the following:

>> **Increases your metabolism.** Aging, muscle loss, and a significant reduction in your metabolic rate all go together. You can fight back by boosting your metabolism through intermittent fasting and muscle-building exercises. Strength training not only can help you manage or lose weight, but it also can increase your metabolism so you burn more calories. Furthermore, a bout of strength training raises your metabolic rate *both* during and after your exercise. This post-exercise calorie burn is scientifically termed excess post-exercise oxygen consumption or EPOC. After a hard workout, your body continues burning calories and fat for up to 48 hours!

>> **Lowers your body fat.** By including strength training in your intermittent fasting program, you have the power to change your body composition by adding to your muscle mass and subtracting disease-promoting body fat.

>> **Increases testosterone levels in men.** Strength training has proven to boost testosterone production in men. To get the largest testosterone boost, experts recommend full-body workouts and lifting heavier weights rather than doing many reps of light weights and shorter rest periods during the workout. Research has also found that strength training workouts may have a bigger effect on testosterone in the evening, suggesting you perform your muscle-building exercises after work.

>> **Protects you from disease.** Strength training is good for the heart. Specifically, strength training has been shown to reduce blood pressure,

increase HDL cholesterol — the good cholesterol — and to reduce blood glucose and insulin levels. Furthermore, some of the leading causes of early death and disability are related to loss of muscle with age. Age-related muscle loss increases risk of the following:

- Arthritis

- Chronic back pain

- Fractures

- Frailty

- Osteoporosis

>> **Reverses age-related cellular decline.** Studies show that just two strength training exercise sessions per week can reverse the damage of muscle decline, a condition called *sarcopenia.* Sarcopenia is characterized by progressive and generalized loss of muscle mass and strength and is correlated with physical disability, poor quality of life, and death.

>> **Extend your life.** Research has shown that having a higher muscle strength index in middle age is among the strongest predictors of a longer lifespan. A muscle strength index is a measure of a person's strength in different parts of the body. For example, hand grip strength is increasingly used by physicians as an indicator of physical wellbeing in the elderly.

>> **Control blood sugar and increase insulin sensitivity.** More muscle means more power to soak up excess blood sugar. Adding to muscle mass also sensitizes muscles to insulin. A study published in the *Journal of Endocrinology & Metabolism* showed that every 10 percent increase in muscle mass results in an 11 percent reduction in risk of insulin resistance and a 10 percent reduction in risk of pre-diabetes.

Planning when and how

You have several choices to consider when planning your strength training workout. If your goal is to gain muscle during your intermittent fasting lifestyle, follow these suggestions:

>> **Calories do count.** For your body to have enough energy to grow your muscles, you need to eat more calories than you burn per day. To gain muscle, you'll need to eat an extra few hundred calories per week. Depending on your intermittent fasting plan of choice, you may need to do the calorie calcs. Check out Chapter 3 for more information.

>> **Time your workouts.** In the case of strength training, schedule your workouts during your eating periods so your nutrition levels are peaked.

>> **Perform strength training geared toward muscle building.** You can choose from many types of weight training schedules and programs. Consult with an exercise professional to construct the program that best fits your lifestyle and goals.

>> **Eat before and after your workout.** Eat a small amount of slow carbohydrates and protein both before and following your workouts (within 30 minutes after your workout) for maximum muscle growth and recovery.

>> **Choose your macros wisely.** A high protein diet isn't necessary to gain muscle. During your eating windows, aim for eating a whole foods, plant-based diet with plentiful amounts of good carbs, plant proteins, and healthy fats.

STRENGTH TRAINING 101

You don't have to be a power lifter to practice strength training. In fact, including it in your exercise plan a couple of times a week, for 30 minutes at a time, while on an intermittent fasting plan can work wonders. Here are some additional pointers about strength training:

- Strength training promotes muscle growth. Examples include the use of free weights, weight machines, resistance bands, or your own body weight.

- The five basic strength training moves are squat, hinge, push, pull, and core work.

- Don't overdo it. Train just two or three times per week to give your muscles time to recover. If you want to train more often, remember that muscle growth occurs during recovery, so switch body parts on alternate days.

- Choose compound multi-joint movement exercises that work multiple major muscle groups, for example, squats, dips, bench press, and deadlifts.

- Make your workouts short and intense rather than long and leisurely.

- Don't waste money on protein supplements that claim to increase muscle mass. (These nutrition allegations aren't scientifically proven.) You can get all the protein you need from regular food.

- If you can afford it, hire a certified personal trainer to help make sure you're doing each exercise correctly, even if it's only for a limited number of sessions. Good advice will increase your gains and reduce your risk of injury.

Destressing with Mindful Exercise

The last type of exercise that compliments your intermittent fasting program is mind-body exercise. Mindful exercise combines body movement, mental focus, and controlled breathing to improve strength, balance, flexibility, and overall health. Creating a mind-body connection means that you use your thoughts to positively influence some of your body's physical responses. Mind-body exercises are helpful in reducing stress, creating a sense of calm, decreasing chronic pain, increasing flexibility, and improving sleep patterns. Examples of mind-body exercise that you can practice daily include:

» Yoga

» Pilates

» Martial arts such as tai chi, tae kwan do, and qi gong

» Muscle relaxation

» Guided imagery

» Rhythmic breathing (controlled breathing exercises)

Of all the mind-body exercises practiced, yoga has become one of the most popular. Here I examine some of the reasons for the rapid rise of yoga afficionados over the last several decades.

Eyeing the many benefits of yoga

Yoga is an ancient practice and tradition developed in India some 5,000 years ago. Today it's a form of exercise that encompasses balance, proper stretching techniques, breathing, meditation, and centering the mind and spirit to foster harmony.

You can choose from many different types of yoga. Every type of yoga has a slightly different definition or interpretation, yet all profess to create a complete system of physical, mental, social, and spiritual development. Try the different styles and find the one that works best for you. Regardless of which form you choose, take note of a few of the multitude of health benefits derived from this type of exercise:

» Improves flexibility and increases range of motion.

» Builds muscle strength.

» Improves muscle tone.

>> Improves balance.

>> Supports joint health.

>> Prevents back pain.

>> Improves breathing techniques.

>> Fosters mental calmness.

Check out the latest edition of *Yoga For Dummies* by Larry Payne and Georg Feuerstein (John Wiley & Sons, Inc.)

Recognizing the art of rhythmic breathing

This mind–body exercise is probably the most effortless exercise, and one you can easily incorporate into your day as a highly effective tool to destress. Rhythmic breathing involves simply taking in long, slow breaths.

Rhythmic breathing is a core part of many meditation and mind–body exercises as it promotes relaxation. Make it a part of your daily exercise routine to complement your intermittent fasting healthy lifestyle program.

To begin one version of rhythmic breathing, follow these steps:

1. **Close your eyes and count slowly to five as you inhale.**

2. **Hold your breath for a few seconds and then count slowly to five as you exhale.**

3. **Pay attention to how your body naturally relaxes.**

   The awareness of breathing draws your focus toward calm. It allows you to remain as relaxed as possible, quieting any stress. Noticing this change will help you to relax even more.

Focus on bettering your breathing techniques. Start your breathing in your nose and be aware of the air moving to your stomach as your diaphragm contracts. Your belly will expand and your lungs will fill with air. You then exhale through your mouth. Make sure to exhale forcefully through your mouth, pursing the lips and making a whoosh sound. This is the most efficient way to breathe, because it pulls down on the lungs, creating negative pressure in the chest and resulting in air flowing into your lungs.

Chapter **15**

Paying Attention to Possible Speed Bumps When Intermittent Fasting

ntermittent fasting can cause side effects, especially if you're not doing it right. In fact, even if done correctly, you'll surely experience some minor bumps in the road, so here is a primer on what to expect. This is also why figuring out which style of intermittent fasting works best for you is so important — a shorter versus longer fasting window or only doing it so many days per week. Refer to Part 3 for the different plans I discuss.

This chapter focuses on common pitfalls encountered during intermittent fasting and suggestions on how to overcome them. If you experience any of them and they don't dissipate after a few weeks or with the suggested remedies, you many need to switch your intermittent fasting protocol to one that works better for you or possibly decide that intermittent fasting simply isn't the right fit.

Handling Hunger Fears

In the beginning of your intermittent fasting journey, you'll definitely feel hungry during your fasting periods. This sensation is perfectly normal. Teaching your body to go 16 hours, 18 hours, or even 24 hours without food takes some practice, and some people might not be capable of eating within a restricted window.

TIP

To help prevent a drop in blood sugar that can trigger irritability during fasting periods, make some dietary adjustments during your food intake period. Ensure you're eating satiating lean protein as well as slow-release fiber-filled complex carbs. Examples of healthy foods rich in slow-releasing carbohydrates are oats, whole grain bread and cereals, bananas, brown rice, quinoa, sweet potatoes, butternut squash, beans, peas, and lentils.

Some people have a fear of hunger, and others develop almost a sense of panic when they start to feel hungry. You can figure out how to accept the feelings and come to terms with the sensation, overcoming your fear. Although doing so may be difficult at first, remember that hunger is your natural guide for meeting your fuel needs. Think of it like a fuel gauge in your car that lets you know when it's time to refuel. Fight back against your fear by repeatedly exposing yourself to hunger during your fasting periods in a safe and controlled way. During this exposure process, you'll discover how to ride out the anxiety and fear until those feelings inevitably pass.

I realize symptoms of hunger aren't pleasant but reassure yourself that they won't hurt you; they're the tools your body uses to alert you that it's time to fuel up. With practice, you'll become more attuned to your hunger cues and know that you can survive and work through them. To overcome the fear of hunger, assure yourself that you'll soon be able to eat, perhaps by reminding yourself that the physiological sensation of hunger isn't dangerous and is time limited. The rewards of sailing through short-term hunger are nothing short of miraculous.

TIP

When you're feeling hangry, try one or more of the suggestions in the section, "Finding Your Stress Relievers," later in this chapter. Remember to breathe.

Curbing Those Cravings

A *food craving* is an intense desire for a specific food. This yearning may seem uncontrollable, and you may think that your longing may not be satisfied until you get that particular food. Cravings are often for junk foods and processed foods high in sugar, salt, and fat. Fortunately, the following tips can help you rein in those cravings:

>> **Remember cravings are time limited.** Experts believe food cravings typically last only 3 to 5 minutes, so remember that and forge though it.

>> **Drink water.** One of the easiest ways to tame food cravings is to fill your stomach with water. Plus, using a straw can help placate oral cravings.

>> **Eat enough protein.** During your eating windows, be sure to eat enough lean protein. Ideally a plant protein is best because you also get a satiating fiber boost. How much is enough? Health experts recommend eating a modest amount of daily protein, far less than the typical American eats. The daily goal for most people is 0.36 grams protein per pound of body weight. That would be just 54 grams for a 150-pound woman, or about one 6-ounce salmon filet.

>> **Chew sugarless gum.** Sugar-free chewing gum is perfectly fine during intermittent fasting and has no effect on blood sugar or insulin levels. Chewing gum is a simple way to keep your mouth busy and has been shown to help reduce both sweet and salty cravings.

>> **Change your environment.** Take a walk around the block, take a long shower, or even call a friend. These things may help distract you long enough for the cravings to subside.

>> **Plan to eat those foods.** Eat the foods you crave, in moderation, during your eating windows. The concept that you aren't depriving yourself can help motivate you.

TIP

People can easily substitute healthier options for typical junk foods. Try some of the suggested alternatives for some of the most common foods that people crave. How do you kick the junk food habit? Don't have it around to tempt you is the best advice. Take the time now to throw the junk food out of the house and replace it with healthier foods. Junk food is loaded with calories, salt, sugar, and/or fat and low in nutrients. Because the food contains unhealthy ingredients and is low in nutrition, nutritionists refer to this type of food as *empty calorie foods* to reflect their lack of nutrients.

Here are some examples of how to substitute healthier, nutrient-dense foods for empty calorie junk foods:

>> **Sugar-laden soft drinks:** Replace with diet sodas, flavored sparkling water, or iced coffee or tea.

>> **Full-fat ice cream:** Replace with frozen yogurts, fat-free ice cream, or fat-free puddings.

> » **Sweets:** Replace with small amounts of dark chocolate or home-baked desserts.

> » **Salty snacks:** Replace with air-popped popcorn seasoned with spray oil and other types of alternative seasonings such as nutritional yeast.

TIP

> *Nutritional yeast* has a cheesy, nutty, savory flavor with a slight salty taste yet is very low in sodium. Nutritional yeast is a species of yeast known as *Saccharomyces cerevisiae,* which is the same type of yeast used to bake bread and brew beer. Nutritional yeast is a great source of B vitamins, minerals, and protein. You can find it at most health food stores.

Igniting Your Energy

In the beginning on your intermittent fasting journey, you may feel fatigued, a natural reaction to curbing your calorie intake. That's because your body is accustomed to using *glucose* — a sugar that comes from the food you eat — for fuel throughout the day. When deprived of food (and, therefore, glucose), you may feel more tired and have less energy than normal.

The good news is that many people feel a serious boost of energy and motivation after they adjust to intermittent fasting. It's a learning experience; as your body adjusts to utilizing alternate fuels, it will get increasingly efficient at burning fat for energy and your energy levels will pick back up. You flip the metabolic switch, which helps improve mood and mental ability and prevent depression. In fact, many people report a higher level of energy when practicing intermittent fasting compared to before.

Here are some tips to help you ignite your energy level:

> » **Exercise.** Fatigue during fasting can also come from being sedentary for too long. Take a brisk walk around the block or do some jumping jacks. These quick bursts of exercise will get your blood flowing and your heart pumping, which will boost your energy level.

> » **Hydrate.** Dehydration is a major cause of fatigue. Adult body composition is more than 60 percent water. Blood is more than 90 percent water, and blood carries oxygen to different parts of the body. That's why drinking enough water can help with energy levels (more oxygen to the working muscles means less fatigue). Practice keeping a huge jug of water by your side during fasting periods and drink up.

- » **Drink a cup a java.** Coffee, without any additives, is a great pick-me-up because caffeine is a proven stimulant. If you can tolerate caffeine, feel free to drink a cup for a quick boost of energy. Some people complain of nausea during fasting periods. If you're drinking too much caffeine, you may become nauseous, so switch to decaffeinated calorie-free drinks. Check out Chapter 8 where I discuss in greater detail how black coffee is a must when intermittent fasting.

- » **Eat slow carbs during your eating windows.** During your fasting window, make sure to eat the slow-digesting healthy carbs that keep your blood sugar on an even keel for long periods of time. They're rich in fiber and, therefore, take longer to digest and cause a slower rise in blood sugar than simple sugars. These fiber-rich slow carbs also prevent you from feeling hungry for hours after eating. Chapter 8 also discusses slow-burning carbs.

WARNING During your fasting periods, you may feel a little tired, hungry, and irritable — but you should never feel sick. If you do, eat a small snack, stop intermittent fasting immediately, and check with your doctor to ensure that intermittent fasting really does work with your body and lifestyle.

Heading Off Headaches

You may experience intermittent fasting headaches, which is one of the most commonly reported side effects. Researchers hypothesize one of the reasons people get headaches during their fasting periods may be due to low blood sugar levels. Yet, research has shown that people with normal blood sugar levels during fasting also may get headaches suggesting that the cause may be something else. With the precise trigger of intermittent headaches currently unknown, pinpointing what's causing yours may not be easy.

Although you may have headaches during your fasting periods, you can plan ahead to both prevent and stop them quickly by doing the following:

- » **Don't withdraw from caffeine.** Caffeine is the world's most widely consumed psychoactive substance. In North America, 90 percent of adults consume caffeine daily. Caffeine increases alertness and decreases fatigue. When the body becomes dependent on caffeine, eliminating it from the diet can cause withdrawal symptoms that typically begin 12 to 24 hours after stopping caffeine. Caffeine withdrawal is a recognized medical diagnosis and can affect anyone who regularly consumes caffeine. The number one side effect of caffeine withdrawal is headaches.

>> **Hydrate.** Dehydration is probably the main cause of fasting headaches. Make sure to drink plenty of water throughout the day during both fasting and nonfasting periods. Even mild dehydration can cause fatigue and headaches. Unfortunately, some people forget to drink water during fasting hours, but going 18 hours a day without enough fluid is a recipe for gastrointestinal disaster. Constipation is another negative side effect of not drinking enough fluids.

>> **Eat nutrient-dense foods to prevent swings in blood sugar.** Having persistent headaches, nausea, or dizziness during intermittent fasting periods could be a red flag that indicates the fasting may be throwing your blood sugar out of whack. To remedy it, make sure the foods you choose to eat during your eating windows are packed with nutrients. A combination of lean protein, healthy high fiber, carbs, and healthy fats will keep your blood sugar level more stable during your fasting windows to prevent possible low blood sugar side effects.

WARNING

Intermittent fasting can cause you to become *hypoglycemic,* a dangerous condition for anyone with insulin or thyroid problems. If you have these issues, stop your fasting immediately and consult with your personal physician. Refer to Chapter 7 for more about hypoglycemia.

>> **Don't break fasts with huge meals.** Depending on what type of intermittent fasting you're following, especially if you're doing any 24-hour fasts such as during Alternate Day intermittent fasting (see Chapter 11) or the Eat-Stop-Eat intermittent fasting plan (refer to Chapter 13), start your refeeding window slowly. Otherwise, a huge meal can leave you feeling fatigued and can cause a rebound headache.

>> **Don't obsess over food during fasting windows.** Try the numerous distraction techniques in the section, "Finding Your Stress Relievers," later in this chapter to help get your mind off food. Stay busy, stay active, but don't overexert yourself during exercise, which can also be a contributing factor for headaches.

Dealing With Scheduling Issues

Fitting all your eating into a 6- or 8-hour window or not eating at all on certain days may be difficult because of your daily schedule. For example, if you have a 9-to-5 job and are following a time-restricted eating plan with your eating window starting at 4 p.m., following this plan may not be feasible if you typically have work-related power lunches. Or, perhaps the only time you can exercise is in the morning and you feel you need to eat before your workout. These types of scheduling conflicts can often make fitting intermittent fasting into your day somewhat difficult.

Intermittent fasting can also make your social life rather challenging. If you're only eating within a certain time period, organizing social events outside of that eating window may be tough. For example, say you've chosen the Warrior plan (see Chapter 10), but you enjoy Sunday brunch with your friends, then you're not going to be able to enjoy Sunday meals and drinks with friends and stay on the plan.

TIP

The best way to avoid intermittent fasting scheduling issues is to choose a plan that works best with your lifestyle *before* you begin. Making a plan around what will fit into your schedule is the best strategy that will prevent feelings of deprivation and keep you motivated.

Finding Your Stress Relievers

Healthy living means spending the time, every single day, to take care of yourself by eating well, exercising, getting enough sleep, and practicing healthful stress management techniques. During your intermittent fasting plan, you may feel stress during your fasting periods.

REMEMBER

Stress is an inevitable part of life, though it needn't get in the way of your healthy lifestyle. Excessive stress that isn't released in a healthful manner can harm you, not only by leaving you prone to developing several diseases, including heart disease and cancer, but also by interfering with your joie de vivre. Here are a few healthy, nonfood-related antistress strategies to keep you on your intermittent fasting track and allow you to live life to the fullest:

>> **Change the environment.** Do something pleasurable or relaxing for a little while such as reading, watching TV, or taking a long, hot shower. Soak in a relaxing bath and let what bothers you go down the drain with the bath water. Creating some alone time to unwind can help you feel calmer and more centered.

>> **Daydream.** Allow yourself a mental time-out. Daydreams can be a calming retreat during a stressful time. Close your eyes, take some deep yoga breaths, and let your mind take you to a relaxing far-off place.

>> **Play cards or a game.** If you enjoy a good game of cards or socializing with friends on the tennis court, then make it a priority in your hectic week to schedule time for recreation. Getting away from work and allowing time for

having fun is a healthy retreat from life's stresses and will take your mind off food if you're in your fasting window.

» **Go for a walk, jog, or bike ride.** Lace up your sneaks, get your heart rate up, and let your problems evaporate with your sweat; exercise is about the healthiest de-stressor there is. Slow your pace if you're fasting and feel less energy than usual.

» **Talk to a friend**. Good friends are hard to find. If you have one, savor the friendship and appreciate the time you spend together. A good friend listens; sharing your thoughts and feelings with a trusted friend is the best medicine for releasing stress and helping you through your fasting periods.

» **Go to a movie, play, or concert.** If you enjoy entertainment, by all means make it a regular occurrence and take the time to enjoy the simple pleasures in life. This activity doesn't have to add stress by hitting your wallet. Many cultural events are free or inexpensive. Check your local newspaper or Facebook for events happening near you.

» **Volunteer.** Volunteering to help others (no matter how large or small the act) can be extremely gratifying and a great way to help yourself as well as others.

» **Get a good night's sleep.** A good night's sleep makes you able to tackle stress more easily. When you're tired, you're less patient and more easily agitated, which can increase resistance to stress. Combining additional stress-lowering tactics to your day can help improve your quality of sleep. On the plus side: Many people report improved sleep patterns while partaking in intermittent fasting regimens.

» **Get a massage.** The power of touch can be extremely therapeutic for both the mind and the body. Reward yourself for even the smallest accomplishment by treating yourself to the human touch — a delicious calorie-free treat — as often as your budget allows.

» **Plant a garden.** Many people find that creating a beautiful flower or vegetable and herb garden is the best way to de-stress. Even better, you can include your homegrown veggies in your meals. You may try participating in a shared community garden or even *container gardening,* growing plants in containers on your patio or balcony.

» **Try relaxation exercises.** Chapter 14 discusses daily relaxation activities like meditation and yoga to soothe your mind and your body. These and other valuable mind-body techniques train you to focus on your breathing and your movements, quieting your mind of the troubles that may be bothering you. Breathing exercises are a simple and highly effective tool to manage stress.

» **Organize something.** Whether it means cleaning the house, organizing your sock drawer, or mowing the lawn, keeping your hands busy and getting something done can bring satisfaction and stress relief to many people.

>> **Read or listen to music.** There's nothing like a good book — the kind you can't put down — to keep your mind occupied and off a stressful situation (or hunger). Enjoying your favorite music, played for your ears only, is also a great way to de-stress. (Or playing an instrument is a fabulous de-stressor.) Some people enjoy listening to audiobooks or relaxation tapes, which can be particularly helpful when you're stressed out while driving in traffic.

>> **Immerse yourself in a creative endeavor.** You may find solace in creative endeavors such as painting, drawing, sculpting, knitting, or woodworking. Taking a class, participating in lifelong learning activities, trying a new hobby, or carving out the time to do something interesting and constructive can take your mind off your worries and is important to fit into your busy schedule.

>> **Pamper yourself.** Get a manicure or pedicure. Pampering yourself can have a tremendous impact on your wellbeing. When you feel good about yourself, your positive self-image will get stronger — and a positive self-image is a valuable tool for healthy living.

>> **Write in your journal.** The physical act of writing down your true feelings on a piece of paper, for your eyes only, can be a powerful way to channel the stress out of your body. Studies have also found that people who are grateful tend to be happier. Journal writing can also help you identify what you're appreciative of in your life. Looking back over these entries can provide you with positive reminders about what's good in your life.

>> **Spend time with an animal.** Yes, dogs are a man's (and woman's) best friend. If you have a pet, savor the unconditional love that flows from animals to humans. Research has proven that giving and receiving affection from animals is a great way to take your mind off your troubles.

>> **Smile and laugh.** Watch your favorite comedy show or movie and escape from your troubles with laughter. Laughter is truly the best medicine. It boosts immunity, lowers stress hormones, relaxes you, adds joy to life, improves moods, and strengthens resilience. A recent study from Norway showed that people with a good sense of humor live longer.

Life is stressful for everyone. The first step in managing stress in a healthy manner is to understand that only when you take care of yourself first can you truly be effective in all the other roles you play in life. Taking more time for self-care may mean saying no to others and realizing that you can't do it all and that trying to do it all and pleasing everyone else is harmful to your health. If you aren't healthy, all areas of your life suffer.

Intermittent fasting can be stressful for some people and may have unpleasant side effects for others. If intermittent fasting causes you stress, try to focus on the two As: adapt and accept. Although the potential side effects may seem intolerable at first, this temporary reaction is just a bump in the road and will dissipate with time.

Chapter **16**

Changing Your Connection with Food

For many people, eating is a distraction from unpleasant feelings, at least in the short run. Turning to food for emotional comfort can cause weight gain and feelings of shame and guilt. If not addressed, it can lead to eating disorders. Becoming aware of your emotional eating patterns is key to a healthy lifestyle intermittent fasting nutrition plan. Other people may not eat from emotions, but they aren't mindful of the food they consume. Eating like that also isn't conducive to good health. In this chapter, you can assess your relationship with food, see if emotional eating and/or mindless eating is a problem for you, and if so, take control.

Assessing Your Relationship with Food

Eating is anything but straightforward for many people. Eating is fuel, providing you with energy to live. Food is life and should be enjoyed. Unfortunately, sometimes the act of eating strays from its purpose and often gets entangled with different emotions, childhood memories, traditional rituals, and cultural ideas. Food becomes far more than fuel, taking on all kinds of meanings — such as solace, reward, punishment, appeasement, and obligation — and depending on the day and your mood, you may end up overeating, undereating, or eating unwisely.

REMEMBER

Developing a healthier relationship with food means first pinpointing where your unhealthy eating patterns are and then working to step out of those patterns and replacing them with healthier behaviors.

Here I help you assess your own relationship with food. If you uncover a problem, then here are some ways to rectify the situation.

Determining what kind of eater you are

Healthy living and long-term weight management involve adopting an active lifestyle and a manageable, nutritionally balanced eating plan. The first step in breaking the chain of unhealthy eating routines is to identify the triggers that start the cycle — patterns, or behavior chains, that you've developed over time and tend to repeat again and again. Knowing the triggers can help you develop behavioral changes that foster a lasting, positive relationship with food.

TIP

To recognize the unhealthy eating situations that affect *you*, regularly record the food you eat, time of day, situations, emotions involved, and the degree of hunger in your journal (Chapter 23 discusses journaling in greater detail). Journaling will allow you to analyze your unhealthy behavior chains and determine where you can break the chain and substitute a healthier alternative.

There are four basic kinds of eaters. Which one best describes you?

>> **Emotional eaters:** You just had a fight with your significant other, and you reach for the bag of chocolate chip cookies. You're sad for whatever reason, and you down a pint of ice cream. You're enjoying a holiday party and overconsume delicious holiday goodies. Like many people, emotional eaters take their mind off whatever they are feeling — sadness, stress, or even happiness — by turning to food. The complexity of emotional eating is the fact that people don't eat because they're hungry. The behavior is oftentimes a compulsion to eat foods that comfort them and help drown the negative emotions. When people eat from emotions, they don't grab something healthy like a carrot for solace — it's usually an entire bag of chips or some-thing similar.

>> **Mindless munchers:** You tend to eat while standing at the refrigerator, driving in your car, streaming your favorite show, or working at your desk. Many people eat when they're distracted, so they have no idea how much they're eating or sometimes even what they're eating.

>> **Carb restrictors:** You're a big fan of fad diets, like Keto, Paleo, or Atkins. You count your carbs, keeping intake to 20 to 100 grams per day. You should know that these types of diets increase your risk of heart disease. These days

carbohydrates have gotten a bad rap. The slew of low-carb diets has made people believe that carbs are the enemy, which is unfortunate because cutting carbs means you're missing out on foods that are important for energy and health. Restricting refined carbs is a wise nutrition move but avoiding good carbs such as whole grains, fruits, and vegetables is not. These foods are loaded with fiber, vitamins, and minerals, and are key for keeping your digestive tract healthy, and helping you feel full.

>> **Healthy eaters:** You've got a healthy relationship with eating, choosing mostly nutritious foods and occasionally indulging without guilt. You eat sitting down at a table with awareness, enjoying every bite of your food and listening to your body's hunger and fullness signals.

TIP

Some people may need the aid of a professional therapist to help them iron out a tough problem or achieve a hefty goal. If you feel that psychological and emotional distress is infringing significantly on your life, seek the aid of a mental health professional.

Taking control of emotional eating behaviors

Figuring out whether you're an emotional eater is important as you pursue an intermittent fasting plan. Ask yourself whether you eat to satisfy your emotions or to diminish your hunger. Emotional eaters consume excessive amounts of food or a specific comfort food item (does chocolate ring a bell for you?) as a response to strong feelings and emotions and/or certain situations. Even when emotional eaters feel full, they're likely to keep eating. Here are some *feelings* and *emotions* that can trigger excessive eating:

>> Anger

>> Anxiety

>> Boredom

>> Depression

>> Fatigue

>> Fear

>> Loneliness

>> Sadness

>> Stress

Here are some *situations* that can trigger excessive eating:

>> Social situations, such as a party or an event

>> Activities such as watching TV or a movie, driving, or reading

>> At a restaurant, after drinking alcohol

>> After thinking negative thoughts such as "I have no willpower"

If you eat more when you're overstressed, you aren't alone. Scientists have proven that many people, especially women, significantly increase their food consumption when they're stressed. Furthermore, stress not only causes people to overeat, but it also affects the type of food many people choose to eat when they're stressed. That food tends to be unhealthy, loaded with sugar and fat. So, fight back against stress overeating by having a prepared plan of action — identify the behavior patterns that have gotten you into trouble in the past and come up with a healthful alternative behavior that will work for you.

TIP

Don't let stress derail your healthy eating habits. Try to include at least one healthy anti-stress strategy into your daily routine. (Flip to Chapters 14 and 15 for lists of healthful de-stressing ideas and activities.) Focus on eating a rainbow of fruits and vegetables, loaded with antioxidants, to help you keep your immune system working at its best.

Breaking Your Behavior Chain

Taking action to break the chain of behavior before the emotional or situational eating sets in is equally important. For example, if streaming your favorite show triggers you to automatically microwave popcorn and a grab a soda, identify that situation and come up with an alternate plan — *before* you tune in. Figure 16-1 illustrates a typical emotional eating behavior chain.

The idea is to break the link in the chain so the behavior is altered. This figure shows several weak links:

>> **At the supermarket:** Don't buy the cookies.

>> **In the kitchen:** When you get back from the supermarket, put the cookies somewhere that you can't reach or don't have access to.

>> **After the argument:** Put on your sneakers and go for a walk or de-stress in a healthful nonfood-related way.

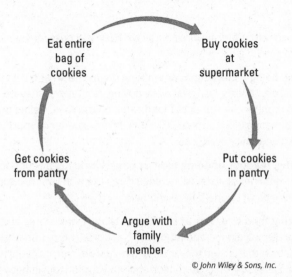

FIGURE 16-1:
An emotional
eating behavior
chain.

TIP

Think about your own behavior chains, which allows you to pinpoint if your emotions are negatively affecting your eating and exercise behaviors. Creating a personal behavior chain allows you to formulate intervention strategies for the future to break the chain.

There are plenty of strategies you can formulate today to put an end to your behavior chain before it starts. Prepare in advance for those sticky situations that may affect your ability to stick to your intermittent fasting plan.

Rearranging your food environment

Think about the locations where you eat or what places trigger you to eat. Do you always snack on chips when you're watching TV? Do you routinely eat the left-overs when cleaning up? Do you eat mindlessly while driving to work? Here are some ways to control your environment and break those habits:

>> **Socializing at parties and other events:** Prepare your strategies ahead of time if the party falls in your eating window (if not, sip on calorie-free drinks). Don't go hungry to social events. Eat a fruit and low-fat yogurt before leaving the house. Alternate alcoholic drinks with sparkling water. Don't stand near the food table. Move around and focus on the conversation, not the food. Make it a potluck. Volunteer to bring a vegetable platter.

>> **Sitting in front of the television:** If it's your eating window, eat your main meal only at the kitchen or dining room table. Plan TV snacks ahead of time in pre-portioned amounts such as 100 calorie microwave popped popcorn, cut-up fruit, or a small bag of baked chips. Air-popped popcorn eaten plain or

seasoned with butter-flavored spray will keep you busy for very few calories and is a good high fiber snack.

>> **Driving, being a passenger, or walking down the street:** If it's your eating window, plan ahead. Don't eat while driving. Not only is it unsafe, but it's too hard to monitor the amount of food eaten on the road. Define one specific place for eating all your meals. Give the dining experience your full attention — sit down and savor every bite.

>> **Studying, reading, or doing tedious paperwork:** Keep your hands busy with a large container of water (sweetened if you like with lemon, a sprig of mint, and a little bit of calorie-free sweetener).

>> **Preparing food or eating at the dinner table:** Drink a large glass of water while preparing dinner, and munch on carrots or cherry tomatoes. Prepare your plate in the kitchen (never serve family style) and limit yourself to one serving. Eat slowly, enjoy each bite, and put your fork down between bites.

>> **Working at the office:** If it's during your eating window, don't get caught off guard. Vending machines are usually loaded with unhealthy snacks, so stay away from them. Bring healthy and easy-to-carry snacks to your workplace. Store healthy foods in the refrigerator or a cold food container.

REMEMBER

Establish a plan to handle situational temptations you regularly encounter. Decide in advance how you'll deal with your weaknesses so that you're in control of the environment and the eating situation.

Changing unhealthy eating behaviors

Change is never easy, especially when it comes to long-established eating behaviors. Here are some tips to help you begin to make healthy eating behavior changes:

>> **Don't strive for perfection.** Denying yourself your favorite foods leads to an all-or-nothing mentality that never works. Set achievable goals. Unrealistic expectations set you up for failure. Slowly change the behaviors that cause you to overeat by identifying and acting on them. Don't forget to include your favorite foods in moderation, slowly eaten using a healthy behavior, savoring every bite.

>> **Try to put a positive spin on things.** Negative thoughts like "I went off my intermittent fasting plan so I'm a failure," or "I can't do this," only serve to undermine your efforts. Take it easy on yourself. A lifetime of poor eating habits takes time and effort to change. Look up inspiring quotes and remind yourself that yes, you can do this!

>> **Get a good night's sleep.** People who don't sleep well are much more prone to overeat. In fact, research has proven that inadequate sleep is linked to obesity. Lack of sleep impairs appetite regulation and blood sugar metabolism and increases blood pressure. Flip to Chapter 6 to get the lowdown on getting a better night's sleep.

Getting a handle on your hunger

Figuring out how to read your body's hunger signals is an important part of healthy eating. Becoming aware of the full spectrum of stomach signals — what constitutes real hunger, what being comfortably full and satisfied feels like, and what the stomach sensations are of being uncomfortably stuffed — will help you to make positive changes in your eating habits. Start now to discover how to differentiate between emotional cravings and true physiological hunger.

Here is the difference between hunger, fullness, and appetite:

>> **Hunger:** *Hunger* is when your body needs to eat. Hunger is the physiological instinct of survival that drives people to feed themselves when the body requires food. Your body tells your brain that your stomach is empty. It's partly controlled by a part of your brain called the *hypothalamus,* your blood sugar level, how empty your stomach and intestines are, and certain hormone levels in your body. Hunger sensations are stomach rumbling, fatigue, lightheadedness, weakness, the shakes, or irritability. Low blood sugar levels and hormone changes that prompt you to eat cause the feeling of hunger.

>> **Fullness:** You eat and then your feel satiated. Fullness is partly controlled by the hypothalamus, your blood sugar, and having food in your stomach and intestines. Your stomach tells your brain that it's full. Normally, this feeling causes you to stop eating and not think about food again for several hours.

>> **Appetite:** *Appetite* is your desire to eat. Appetite is psychological, the desire for food. Sometimes hunger triggers appetite, but many times appetite is due to cravings, habits, the availability of food, or other social and emotional factors (such as happiness, boredom, sadness, anxiety, and so on). Even seeing and smelling food (like strolling through the mall with the pretzel scent wafting through your nostrils) can trigger your desire to eat.

TIP

Eating based on appetite alone rather than actual hunger can result in eating more than you need. Discovering how to eat food based on hunger (rather than emotions) and stopping eating when you're full are important components of a healthy relationship with food.

Diving into Mindful Eating

Eating has become a mindless endeavor in today's fast-paced, multitasking distracted world, which can be problematic because it takes your brain up to 20 minutes to realize you're full. To battle this unhealthy eating behavior, the concept of mindful eating has evolved. *Mindful eating* is a technique based on mindfulness, a Buddhist concept, that helps people become aware of their thoughts, feelings, and physical sensations related to eating. People can distinguish between their appetite and physical hunger. It also increases recognition of food-related triggers and gives people the freedom to choose how to respond to them. The following sections delve deeper into mindful eating and explain how you can include it in your intermittent fasting plan.

WEB EXTRAS

The Center for Mindful Eating is a is a member-supported, nonprofit international organization. The organization's mission is to help people achieve a balanced, respectful, healthy and joyful relationship with food and eating. Check out www.thecenterformindfuleating.org for more information.

Practicing mindful eating techniques

Mindful eating is a powerful tool to regain control of your eating. Combined with the practice of intermittent fasting and eating a whole, plant-based diet, you have the perfect trifecta for living your best life. To help you incorporate mindful eating into your life, check out some of these principles and practices:

>> **Identifying your hunger cues.** Figuring out how to identify hunger cues can help you differentiate between hunger and appetite. Different degrees of hunger exist, so to differentiate yours, you can use a hunger scale (see Figure 16-2) where you number your degrees of hunger throughout the day in your journal (Chapter 23 discusses journaling in greater depth). This simple exercise will enable you to understand what real hunger feels like and can help you tune back in to your body and decide whether your desire to eat comes from real hunger or other reasons. Try this for a few days so you can figure out how to recognize the true hunger sensation during your intermittent fasting journey.

>> **Recognizing degree of fullness.** Assessing your level of satiety and stopping eating before you're extremely full is another exercise in mindful eating training. You can also use your hunger scale to assess degrees of fullness.

1	2	3	4	5	6	7	8	9	10
Starving, dizzy	Very hungry, irritable	Fairly hungry, stomach growling	Getting hungry, thinking of food	Neutral, no hunger feelings	Slightly full, satisfied	Full, slightly un-comfortable	Stuffed	Very un-comfortable	Painfully full, feeling sick

FIGURE 16-2: A hunger scale.

>> **Slowing down your eating.** Slower eating is the key to easier weight loss or maintenance and greater satisfaction with meals. One method nutritionists often recommend to help people stop gobbling down food at a rapid pace, without even tasting it, is to put your fork down between bites. Another idea is to eat with chopsticks. Focus on chewing; some dietitians suggest chewing your food a minimum of 32 times per bite to prolong your eating experience.

REMEMBER

Mindful eating helps you restore your attention to the food and slow down, making eating an intentional act instead of an automatic one. What's more, by increasing your recognition of physical hunger and fullness cues, you're able to distinguish between emotional and true, physical hunger.

Reviewing the habits of healthy eaters

Every day, you make choices about the food you eat and your lifestyle. Healthy eaters are people who eat a variety of foods that provide the nutrients needed to maintain health, feel good, and have energy. These nutrients include protein, carbohydrates, fat, water, vitamins, and minerals. Healthy eaters choose their food wisely and eat a more whole, plant-centered diet. From reducing disease risk to improving brain function and fitness, a healthy diet is vital for every aspect of life. There is also the psychological side of healthy eating. Healthy eaters have figured out how to have a beneficial relationship with food.

Healthy eaters have many of the following habits in common:

>> **Tune in to hunger and fullness.** Healthy eaters are aware of the physiological sensations of hunger and respect them. They're unafraid of feeling some hunger between meals. Mild hunger is a good thing. After all, it's a sign that you're not overeating. Teach yourself to appreciate hunger pangs as a natural part of life and as a sign that you're a healthy eater. Healthy eaters don't eat from emotions and external cues (appetite) but instead from true hunger. Healthy eaters stop eating when they're satisfied, not stuffed. Unhealthy eaters have stopped listening to body signals of hunger and fullness.

>> **Be assertive at restaurants.** Healthy eaters are politely picky at restaurants. Most restaurant food is loaded with salt, fat, and calories. Healthy eaters ask the server how foods are prepared and order menu items that are baked, broiled, roasted, seared, poached, or steamed.

>> **Shop savvy at the supermarket.** Healthy eaters take their time food shopping. They read labels and know what foods they're buying and eating.

>> **Garden and attend farmers' markets often.** Healthy eaters know that homegrown food is better for your health and the environment. They practice eating more locally grown foods and eat sustainably.

>> **Practice moderation.** Healthy eaters don't torture themselves over a bite of chocolate or always look for the lowest calorie recipe. They enjoy all kinds of foods in moderation, without guilt.

>> **Be aware of food safety.** Healthy eaters keep the refrigerator and freezer at proper temperatures, defrost food in the refrigerator, and know how to prevent cross-contamination.

5

Intermittent Fasting Made Easy: Eating, Shopping, and Cooking

Organize your kitchen to make it your fountain of health.

Navigate the grocery store and stock your kitchen and pantry for success.

Peruse the healthiest and definitely tastiest diet to add to your intermittent fast.

Create delicious and easy-to-make intermittent-fasting-friendly recipes.

Chapter **17**

Adding the Mediterranean Diet to Your Intermittent Fasting Plan

At the beginning of every new year, *U.S. News & World Report*, the global authority in rankings and consumer advice, releases its annual assessment of the year's best diets. In 2020, for the third consecutive year, the Mediterranean Diet remained at the No. 1 spot. The diet also took the top spot in four other lists:

» Best Diets for Healthy Eating

» Easiest Diets to Follow

» Best Diets for Diabetes

» Best Plant-Based Diets

Why all the excitement? The Mediterranean Diet is easy to follow, the food tastes great, and the lifestyle is good for your health. For the millions of people making health-related resolutions for the New Year — or any time of year, for that matter — now's the time to try this popular and delicious and nutritious Mediterranean-style eating regimen. I urge you to enjoy a long and healthy life by following the Mediterranean lifestyle — scientifically proven to be the world's healthiest (and tastiest) diet. This chapter explores what has been proven to be the healthiest way of eating and living for disease prevention, anti-aging and longevity.

The Mediterranean Diet isn't a fad diet or quick scheme to lose weight, but rather a healthy way of eating and living that will last a lifetime — the perfect accompaniment to your intermittent fasting plan. The Mediterranean Diet has long been celebrated as the gold standard of healthy diets for its highly palatable nature and favorable impact on the prevention of chronic diseases, promotion of greater longevity, and quality of life. You want to incorporate a diet into your lifestyle that's sustainable; research about the Mediterranean Diet has shown it provides the healthiest long-term benefits.

The foundation of the Mediterranean Diet is vegetables, fruits, herbs, nuts, beans, olive oil, and whole grains. Meals are built around these whole, plant-based foods. Although researchers aren't completely sure which components of the diet provide the greatest health benefits, the takeaway is that eating a variety of nutritious unprocessed and minimally processed foods work together in synergy. So, in a nutshell (yes, nuts are a component of this diet) I encourage you to incorporate the foods that comprise the diet into your intermittent fasting plan, as well as becoming more physically active, so that you can begin to reap the massive health benefits that this lifestyle has to offer.

For more in-depth information about the Mediterranean Diet and more than 150 recipes, check out the latest edition of *Mediterranean Diet Cookbook For Dummies* by Meri Raffetto (John Wiley & Sons, Inc.).

Incorporating the Mediterranean Diet into Your Intermittent Fasting Plan

Intermittent fasting isn't a diet; it's a pattern of eating. The focus of an intermittent fast is not on *what* you eat but *when* you eat. Adding the Mediterranean Diet to your intermittent fasting plan is simple: When you eat, you eat an abundance of plant foods: fruits, vegetables, whole grains, legumes, and nuts. In addition, extra-virgin olive oil (EVOO) is the main fat and fish is emphasized as a protein source, which is an excellent way to obtain heart-healthy omega-3 fat. The Mediterranean Diet also offers heart-healthy monounsaturated fatty acids, inflammation-fighting phytochemicals, gut-friendly prebiotic fiber, and a wealth of vitamins, minerals, and antioxidants.

Here are some easy ways to start living the Mediterranean lifestyle:

>> Make authentic EVOO your main fat for cooking, salad dressings, and dipping bread. Use avocado as a spread.

>> Eat lots of fresh vegetables every day, especially deeply colored green, orange, red, and purple produce.

>> Season food with herbs, wine, citrus, vinegars, and garlic in lieu of salt.

>> Eat 100 percent whole grain products every day.

>> Eat seafood *at least* twice a week (to obtain lean protein and healthy omega-3 fat).

>> Eat some fresh fruit every day.

>> Eat a handful of nuts and some flaxseeds or chia seeds (plant omega-3 fat) every day.

>> Eat legumes (beans, peas, or lentils) every day.

>> Eat a small amount of yogurt (either fat-free dairy or soy) daily.

>> Drink a glass of red wine with dinner (if your healthcare professional gives you the okay).

>> Walk a minimum of 30 minutes a day (aim for achieving 10,000 steps) and strength train twice a week (for healthy bones) — Chapter 14 discusses more about exercise.

>> Enjoy your meals, savoring every bite and sharing the experience with family and friends.

WEB EXTRAS

For an in-depth description of the Mediterranean Diet plus myriad tips on following the Mediterranean lifestyle, visit my website at `www.mediterranean nutritionist.com/`.

EAT LIKE YOU'RE IN CRETE

If you were to visit Crete, more than likely you'd sit down at a seaside restaurant to a mouthwatering meal of grilled fish right off the boat, perhaps a thick, juicy, halibut steak, seasoned with nothing more than a drizzle of authentic EVOO, fresh garlic, a squeeze of lemon juice, and accompanied by the ubiquitous green veggies. Or, perhaps you may savor an exquisitely succulent fish stew, overflowing with the bounty of the sea, such as clams, fish fillet, and scallops simmered in a garlic, olive oil, and tomato-based stock, a meal that will give you all the protein you need with half the calories and twice the taste of beef.

When you eat like you're in Crete, imagine yourself sitting down to dinner over a leisurely meal and enjoying delicious, fresh, and artfully prepared food, slowly savoring the joy of your Mediterranean food — a far cry from mindlessly gobbling down your food behind your steering wheel or in front of your computer screen. Eating like a Mediterranean is as much lifestyle as it is a diet.

Grasping the Laws on Lean Protein

The typical, disease-promoting Western diet is characterized by high intakes of trans and saturated fats, full-fat dairy, refined sugars, refined and highly processed vegetable oils, sodium, and processed foods. That's in stark contrast to the Mediterranean Diet, a whole, plant-based diet filled with fresh fruits and vegetables, nuts, olive oil, and whole grains that avoids red and processed meats, full-fat dairy, trans and saturated fats, and refined sugars.

One of the easiest ways to cut down on your intake of disease-causing types of bad fats is to change your protein source. A simple strategy is to avoid eating beef. By omitting just one food from your diet, *you* can have a significant impact on climate change. Livestock accounts for roughly 15 percent of the world's greenhouse gases each year. That's approximately the same amount as the emissions from all the cars, trucks, airplanes, and ships combined in the world today. Cows alone are responsible for most of the livestock's contribution, releasing huge amounts of methane. Methane is at least 28 times as destructive as carbon dioxide when it comes to heating the atmosphere. In fact, cows make a massive contribution to the planet's greenhouse gas emissions. Cattle devour more land and water and causes more environmental damage than any other single food product.

The following sections focus on what kind of protein you should eat and why.

Eat more plant and fish protein

The mantra for wanting to preserve your health and the health of the planet: Eat more plant protein and less animal protein. One way to do this is to narrow your choices. Choose mostly vegetable protein and add in a little fish and very occasionally, skinless poultry. That's it — cut back on all other animal sources of protein especially bad fat-laden red and processed meats. Choose mostly plant proteins, keep the portions of your lean animal protein relatively small, and bake, broil, or poach the food rather than bread and fry to incorporate the best protein nutrition strategy into your life.

The bottom line is that when adding protein to your diet, the plant-fish Mediterranean habit provides the most powerful protection against disease and is an easy and tasty way to ensure that you're enjoying the right amount and type of protein to make a difference in living better and eating for life, the Mediterranean way. Include some protein at each meal and also try to include a serving of yogurt (preferably soy) daily. Choose your protein wisely using the plant-fish concept in Table 17-1 and eat for life the Mediterranean way.

TABLE 17-1   **Protein Choices — Mediterranean Style**

Primary Protein: Plants	Secondary Protein: Marine Protein
Beans	Salmon
Peas	Tuna
Lentils	Sardines
Soy	Shrimp
Nuts	Clams
Whole Grains	Scallops

REMEMBER

For a long and healthy life choose mostly plant and fish sources of protein most of the time, but that doesn't mean you have to give up meat completely. If you do choose to eat poultry, red meat, or pork, pick the leanest cuts; choose only skinless poultry; bake, broil, or poach; eat it only occasionally; and resist the urge to make it the centerpiece of your meal. Take your Mediterranean Diet and incorporate a little Asian. Think Chinese food, where the bulk of the meal is usually carbohydrate (vegetables and rice, albeit white rice; just replace with brown rice) and the animal protein is more like a condiment.

And no need to worry about getting a complete protein in with your plant foods. The term *complete protein* refers to amino acids, the building blocks of protein. There are 20 different amino acids that can form a protein and nine that your body can't produce on its own (also known as *essential amino acids*). To be considered complete, a protein must contain adequate amounts of all nine essential amino acids. Despite the fact that only a handful of plant proteins are considered complete, most nutritionists believe that plant–based diets contain such a wide variety of amino acid profiles that even vegans are virtually guaranteed to get all their essential amino acids in every day.

For vegans and vegetarians: Focus on plant protein

However, if you want to eat a complete plant protein without eating animal protein, here is a list of plant proteins that contain enough of all the essential amino acids in one food:

>> **Amaranth:** An ancient grain also a pseudo-cereal, meaning that it's not technically a cereal grain like wheat or oats

>> **Buckwheat:** From the plant *Fagopyrum esculentum,* cultivated for its grain-like seeds

>> **Chia seeds:** From the flowering plant *Salvia hispanica,* a species of flowering plant in the mint family, grown for its edible seeds

>> **Ezekiel bread:** A flourless bread made from sprouted grains

>> **Hemp seeds or hearts:** Seeds from the plant *Cannabis sativa*

>> **Nutritional yeast:** A deactivated yeast, often a strain of *Saccharomyces cerevisiae*

>> **Quinoa:** An ancient whole grain that technically isn't a cereal grain, but a pseudo-cereal

>> **Soybeans:** Including tofu, tempeh, and edamame

>> **Spirulina:** A type of blue-green algae

Add healthy fish protein

When you do eat seafood, keep in mind certain factors to ensure the fish you eat is healthy for you and for the environment. That means consuming fish that's both low in mercury and sustainably caught. Choosing seafood that is both healthy and sustainable can be tricky. The good news is that tools are available to help you make smart seafood choices more easily.

WEB EXTRAS The easiest way to make the best seafood choices is to check the Monterey Bay Aquarium's Seafood Watch guide at www.seafoodwatch.org. The site has a guide that uses a rigorous, science-based process to grade seafood choices as best choices, good alternatives, or seafood to avoid.

Making Extra-Virgin Olive Oil (EVOO) Your Main Fat

No doubt about it, fat makes food taste great. Don't believe the hype that "butter is back" and is healthy. Despite what the media has led people to believe, butter is *not* a heart-healthy food. Butter is rich in saturated fat and dietary cholesterol, two types of fatty substances that have proven to raise the risk of coronary artery disease. Butter is a major source of saturated fat intake in the United States. Instead, for your health and your taste buds, switch from animal fat to the healthiest vegetable fat out there, EVOO and make EVOO your main fat — the core of the Mediterranean Diet.

Olive oil is actually a fruit juice because it's made from crushing and pressing a whole fruit (olive) — pits and all — as opposed to a seed (such as rapeseed, the source of canola oil) or a vegetable (corn). In fact, olive oil is the most widely consumed fruit juice in the world. Because olives are a fruit, they provide a large amount of plant antioxidants called *polyphenols,* which are scarce in other oils derived from seeds or vegetables. The minimal processing of EVOO makes for a healthier fat due to the more natural state of the plant oil and the lack of excess heat and chemicals used to process it. Moreover, olive oil is one of the few oils that retains the natural flavor, antioxidants, vitamins, minerals, and other healthful components of the vegetable, seed, or in this instance the ripe olive fruit.

The problem is that that bottle of olive oil in your pantry, the one you bought for its purported health benefits and to help you adhere to the much revered and seductive Mediterranean lifestyle, is most likely a scam. Authentic EVOO, the kind that is truly a healing superfood, is hard to find in the marketplace. In fact, 7 out of 10 bottles of extra virgin olive oil sold in a U.S. supermarket were fake, according to a study performed by the UC Davis Olive Center.

REMEMBER Olives are a fruit. Authentic EVOO is like fresh-squeezed fruit juice — seasonal and never better than the first few weeks it was made. *Remember:* true EVOO is *extremely perishable*!

TIPS FOR BUYING EVOO

Making sure you're buying real, exceptionally healthful, and unadulterated EVOO is important. The following list helps you skirt the scams so you purchase authentic EVOO from reputable producers, which ideally fosters greater consumption of EVOO, a vital, health-promoting food:

- Buy oil in a dark glass or other containers that protect against light and air. Keep it well sealed and store in a cool, dark place away from heat and sunlight.

- Choose a small bottle or can and replenish it often.

- Select only labels that read *extra virgin*, not *pure, light oil, olive oil,* or *pomace olive oil.*

- Buy only oil with a *harvest date* stamped on it to ensure freshness.

- Avoid bottling scams. Watch out for phrases like *packed in Italy* or *bottled in Italy*; they don't mean that the oil was made in Italy. Only buy oil whose precise point of production — a specific mill is listed.

- Buy oil with the highest polyphenol content (above 500), which is an important indicator of the oil's range of health-giving characteristics.

- Look for a free fatty acid level (FFA) of 0.2 percent or lower, FFA and peroxides at well below 10 meq/kg.

- Buy oil with a certification seal such as PDO and PGI, Australian Olive Association, the California Olive Oil Council, and the Association 3E.

- Avoid bargain prices; producing a genuine extra virgin oil is expensive (and worth every penny)!

- Choose authentic EVOO highest in polyphenol content and with the most recent harvest date. To ensure your oil is authentic, make sure to buy it from a single source reputable seller. My favorite online site for buying the real thing is Seasons. (No need to buy organic because olives are grown with little or no pesticides.) Check out http://seasonstaproom.com and click on "Super Premium Varietal Extra Virgin Olive Oil."

Keeping Those Grains Whole

You may be like many others who are fearful of eating carbs because you think they're fattening. That's unfortunate, because if you cut back on carbs, and especially the good carbs, you automatically reduce your intake of one of the top sources of fiber. Whole grains are carbs, the healthy good carbs — packed with nutrition. The U.S. government recommends that you make at least half of your daily grains whole (which comes to at least three servings of whole grains per day), but most Americans — 96 percent in fact — fall woefully short of that goal. The truth is most Americans fail to get in even one serving of whole grains per day, although consumers are completely unaware of how much they're eating. Surveys find that 60 percent respond that they feel like they're getting enough whole grains. That's a huge gap for Americans.

This is a problem because whole grains are a high-fiber food, and high-fiber diets, such as the Mediterranean Diet, prevent a host of diseases including heart disease, certain types of cancer, and obesity, and may even extend life.

These sections take a closer look at the whole grain and help you select whole grains when you're shopping.

Examining a whole grain

Natural whole grains contain three botanically defined parts:

>> **Bran:** The *bran* is the multilayered outer skin of the kernel. Most of the healthy disease-fighting phytochemicals are concentrated in the bran layer as are most of the minerals and fiber.

>> **Endosperm:** The *endosperm* is the energy-containing center, largely starch, that is the germ's food supply.

>> **Germ:** The *germ* resides inside the endosperm; it's the nutrient storehouse, containing healthy fats, vitamins, minerals, and some protein.

Eat the whole seed, or *kernel*, with the three parts intact — the entire complex — and you're eating a complete whole grain that packs a powerful nutritional punch. Refined grains have had the bran and most of the germ portions removed, so you're basically left eating just the endosperm of the rice kernel when you choose white rice over brown. When you remove the germ and bran layers, you lose most of the fiber, B vitamins, vitamin E, healthy fats, and about 75 percent of the phytochemicals and antioxidants. Figure 17-1 illustrates the three original parts of a whole grain.

When food manufacturers eliminate the bran and germ of the rice kernel in processing, the grain is stripped of much of its disease-fighting potential. In fact, refining wheat, another type of grain, removes most of the naturally occurring vitamins, minerals, and other nutrients including the lion's share of wheat's potent polyphenol antioxidant called *ferulic acid.*

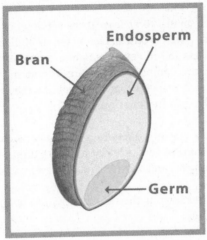

FIGURE 17-1:
A grain — the
bran, germ, and
endosperm.

Source: Whole Grains Council,
`www.wholegrainscouncil.org.`

TIP

"Three is key" is a common saying among registered dietitians. Aim for eating three whole grain servings in a day or approximately 48 grams of whole grain each day (unless it's a fasting day). This recommendation is based on the scientific evidence that people who eat at least this much are less likely to develop heart disease.

Finding a whole grain food

The easiest way to spot a whole grain food is to look for 100 percent of the grain listed on the ingredient list to be whole. For example, the only grain in a tin of steel-cut oatmeal is *whole* oats. Be wary that many foods, such as breads, crackers, and ready-to-eat breakfast cereals, are made with a combination of whole and refined grains, making it difficult to evaluate its whole grain status. That's why the Oldways Whole Grains Council, a nonprofit organization working to increase whole grains consumption, developed the Whole Grain Stamp program.

DIFFERENTIATING BETWEEN WHITE AND BROWN RICE

Choose the white variety and you swallow a fiber-less bundle of starch — fortified with iron and some B vitamins — but still missing many key nutrients located in the bran or outer fibrous layer covering the rice kernel that has been removed during refining. Choose the brown rice and you're eating a grain the way Mother Nature packaged it, a wonderful source of an array of natural vitamins and minerals, antioxidants, and fiber — nutrients that are mostly lost in the refining process.

The program has three different Stamps:

» 100% Stamp

» 50% + Stamp

» Basic Stamp

Manufacturers can apply to use the "100% Whole Grain Stamp" on food packages meaning that the product provides one serving of whole grains (16 grams) per serving. These Stamps, found on more than 13,000 products in 63 countries, can help you choose whole grain products with confidence. Figure 17-2 shows what the Whole Grain Stamps looks like. When shopping, preferentially choose products exhibiting the 100 percent Whole Grain Stamp.

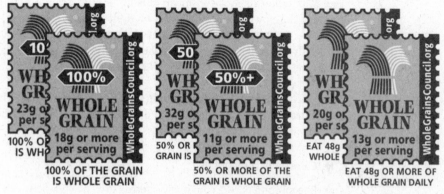

FIGURE 17-2:
Whole Grain
Stamps.

100% OF THE GRAIN IS WHOLE GRAIN

50% OR MORE OF THE GRAIN IS WHOLE GRAIN

EAT 48g OR MORE OF WHOLE GRAIN DAILY

Source: Whole Grains Council, www.wholegrainscouncil.org.

To find whole grains in the grocery store, take the time to remember their names. Common varieties include

» Amaranth

» Barley

» Brown rice

» Buckwheat

» Corn

» Millet

» Popcorn

» Quinoa

- » Whole-grain barley

- » Whole oats/oatmeal

- » Whole-wheat couscous

- » Wild rice

- » 100 percent whole-wheat flour

- » 100 percent whole-grain bread

Powering Up with Plants

The foundation of Mediterranean cuisine is built around plants. If you want to harness the power of antioxidants to fight disease and aging, you need to eat plants — and lots of them. Plant foods have the ability to prevent illness and heal, especially deep, dark greens drenched in olive oil — heart and blood pressure medicine, Mediterranean style — taken on a daily basis.

Plant foods are loaded with plant chemicals (*phytochemicals*). Thousands of phytochemicals have been identified, and those that have been studied the most have been divided into three major groups:

- » Carotenoid compounds,

- » Phenol compounds, commonly referred to as polyphenols

- » Organosulfur compounds

Tap into this natural medicine chest by filling your plate with phytochemical plant foods.

When phytochemicals are consumed, their antioxidant and anti-inflammatory properties work in concert to mop up free radicals — the dangerous molecules that propagate inflammation. But don't be fooled by what drug companies tell you; taking dietary supplements consisting of isolated pure antioxidant plant compounds doesn't have the same health-promoting effects as eating a plant-based diet.

A whole foods plant-based diet of home-cooked and less highly processed foods — in other words a Mediterranean-type approach — can help you lower your risk for chronic disease, manage your weight, and boost your energy. You may be new to the concept of what a whole food, plant-based diet is, so here are a few tips to get you started:

>> **Eat lots of vegetables.** Fill your plate with a rainbow of brightly colored vegetables at mealtime. Enjoy vegetables as a snack with hummus, salsa, or guacamole.

>> **Eat nuts and seeds often.** Nuts and seeds are also antioxidant polyphenol powerhouses. Nuts have impressive effects on cholesterol and triglyceride levels — lowering both bad LDL cholesterol and dangerous triglyceride levels. Nuts have been shown to promote weight loss rather than contribute to weight gain. Nuts are high in healthy fats and fiber and are a great source of several nutrients, including vitamin E, magnesium, and selenium. Eat as a snack, use a nut spread as a sandwich spread, add some to salads, and drink almond milk to get in some daily nuts.

>> **Choose healthy plant fats.** Fats in olive oil, nuts and nut butters, seeds, and avocados are exceptionally healthy choices.

>> **Build your meals with plants.** Create healthy dishes using legumes (beans, peas, or lentils), whole grains, and vegetables.

>> **Eat fresh fruit for dessert.** A ripe, juicy peach and a refreshing slice of watermelon will satisfy your sweet tooth without the calories and additives of processed desserts. For example, choose a crisp apple over a slice of apple pie.

>> **Choose frozen produce.** Despite what you may have heard, frozen produce is really healthy and typically retains more nutrients than fresh produce. You'll get just as much nutrition — for a whole lot less money — by buying frozen foods instead of fresh. Just make sure that you buy single ingredient frozen produce (no additives). For example, a bag of frozen broccoli florets should have a single ingredient, broccoli, on the ingredient list. Check out Chapter 18 for a tutorial on interpreting Nutrition Facts label lingo.

>> **Buy fresh and local.** Buy plant foods directly from local producers by visiting your farmers' market, joining a community-supported agriculture (CSA) association, or buying directly from a local farm.

Chapter 18

Going Grocery Shopping, Healthfully

L ife is fast, fast, fast. With the onslaught of information bombarding you on a daily basis, it's important for your wellbeing to figure how to cull back what's important and let the rest go. This strategy is particularly sage advice when navigating the supermarket aisles. The never-ending barrage of contradictory nutrition advice and the myriad food choices can make a trip to the supermarket a harrowing experience.

You may feel constantly bombarded with information regarding technology, medical findings, and current events, which can be overwhelming to say the least. I hope to ease your anxiety a bit. Healthy eating begins at the grocery store by discovering how to choose great-tasting, nutrient-dense foods. The typical supermarket carries more than 50,000 food items. To help you make sense of the supermarket maze, this chapter addresses the ways you can make the most nutritious food choices to accompany your intermittent fasting plan.

Finding Your Way around the Supermarket

Being able to navigate your grocery store is so important when you're shopping for healthful and fresh foods. In the following sections I help you put together a plan of attack before you go shopping and then walk you through a typical grocery store, directing you to the areas where you can find the right kinds of food for your intermittent fasting plan (as well as what areas to avoid).

Shopping with a plan

Good nutrition starts at the grocery store. Here are some savvy supermarket shopping tips:

TIP

>> **Prepare ahead.** Make your shopping list before you go. Survey your refrigerator, freezer, and pantry and write down on a notepad or make a note in your phone what you need. If possible, plan in advance what meals you'll be eating (or not eating) on each day, beforehand so you can shop for the recipes you'll be making. This list will keep you focused on buying the healthier food options. Plus, this simple strategy will save you time, money, and pounds on the scale. Don't deviate from the list unless it's for extra fruits and vegetables.

   Furthermore, making a shopping list beforehand also helps you get in and out of the store more efficiently, carrying only what's on your list. With a healthy shopping list in hand, you'll be less likely to make spontaneous, unhealthy food purchases.

>> **Shop on a full stomach.** Don't go to the supermarket during your fasting periods. People who are ravenous when they go to a supermarket are often tempted to buy impulsively. If you're super hungry, you may not be as discerning in your healthy nutrition choices. If you're hungry and you're in your eating window, pick up a container of pre-cut fresh fruit and nibble on it while you shop.

>> **Choose the healthy frozen foods.** Frozen fruit and vegetables are highly nutritious. Just be sure to go for the "single ingredient" frozen foods; for example, if you're buying peas, the ingredient list should read "peas."

>> **Think fresh.** Fresh food, food that hasn't been processed, is your best bet for good nutrition. Processed foods tend to be much higher in unhealthy additives such as salt, sugar, and bad fats.

>> **Once in the store, take your time.** Go shopping when you have plenty of time. This way you can use the time to analyze and compare food labels. After you get familiar with the differences in brands and products offered, you won't need to spend as much shopping.

Analyzing where everything is located in the supermarket

Supermarkets across the board are laid out the same way. Whole and fresh foods tend to be located on the perimeter of the supermarket, whereas the aisles have the more processed foods. Figure 18-1 depicts a typical supermarket layout. Most importantly, when you're shopping, stick to the perimeter of the store. The perimeter is where you'll find the fresh produce, lean meats/chicken/fish, and fat-free dairy. Only venture into the aisles to pick up low-sodium canned beans, tomato products, whole grain breads, cereals, pasta (don't forget popcorn kernels), water-packed tuna, nut butters, extra-virgin olive oil, oil sprays, and vinegars.

FIGURE 18-1: Shop the perimeter of the supermarket for the freshest foods.

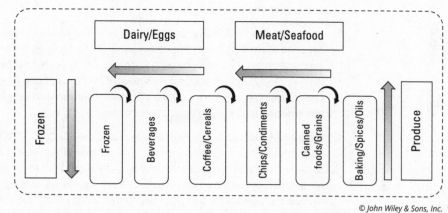

© John Wiley & Sons, Inc.

One technique that can help you make better choices is to shop by food groups. Divide your list into these six categories:

TIP

>> **Fruits and vegetables:** Fresh fruits and vegetables are the basis of a healthy diet. They're packed with antioxidants, fiber, vitamins, and minerals. Eating lots of this group will benefit your health and your weight and will help prevent chronic disease.

Opt for a painter's palette of colors of fruits and vegetables. Remember, the darker the color, the greater the nutrient value. Always choose richly colored fruits and vegetables over pale-colored ones. Select a cancer-fighting cruciferous vegetable like broccoli over celery, spinach over iceberg lettuce, and red grapes over green. Dark-hued produce contains the most disease-fighting antioxidants. Unfortunately, most Americans' intake of dark green and cruciferous vegetables is far too low. I suggest you try a new fruit or vegetable each week in your shopping list. Experiment with new flavors and combinations of food to get even more vitamins and minerals.

>> **Whole grains:** Rich in fiber, B vitamins, and complex carbohydrates, whole grains are essential for energy production and health maintenance. Opt for whole-grain breads, pastas, crackers, and rice. Choose breads/cereals with at least 3 grams of fiber and less than 3 grams of fat per serving. Refer to the section, "Knowing How to Read Labels," later in this chapter for help deciphering the packaging.

>> **Calcium-rich products:** This group contains important sources of calcium, protein, and vitamin D, nutrients that are essential for keeping your bones healthy and strong. Choose fat-free or low-fat dairy products. Fat-free, calcium-rich products have the same amount of calcium as full-fat dairy products but are minus the artery-clogging saturated fat. Fat-free Greek yogurt packs a powerful calcium punch. If you prefer not to eat dairy, plant milks and yogurts are also excellent choices such as almond milk, soy milk and yogurt, and oat milk.

>> **Lean proteins:** This food group provides excellent sources of protein, iron, zinc, and vitamin B12 — all important nutrients for building the proteins that your body requires. Seafood is rich in omega-3 fatty acids, and beans are high in fiber. Always opt for lean, skinless poultry over meat. Egg whites give you a perfect amino acid profile (called a *high quality protein*) with very few calories (the white from one large egg contains a mere 17 calories).

>> **Nuts and seeds:** Rich in polyunsaturated and monounsaturated fats (the good ones), vitamin E, and selenium, nuts are a delicious, heart-healthy food. Because nuts are high in calories and fat (albeit, good fat) enjoy them in moderation or you'll pay at the scale. Choose natural dry-roasted (unsalted) almonds or walnuts for two great sources of healthy fats. Chia seeds are shelf stable, contain loads of fiber and healthy fat, and are a complete protein source.

>> **Fats and sweets:** Rich in calories, food items containing excessive amounts of fat and/or sugar should be consumed judiciously for better health and to prevent weight gain. If you're going to include a sweet treat as part of your intermittent fasting eating plan, look for small, individually wrapped 100-calorie or less packaged sweets. Opt for low-fat condiments, sauces, or salad dressings. Choose healthy oils such as extra-virgin olive oil (EVOO) and oil sprays.

Organizing your shopping cart

You can also organize your cart for food safety and efficiency. Here are the three factors to keep in mind while pushing your cart through the aisles:

>> **Choose cold and frozen foods last.** Add the cold and frozen items to your cart at the end of your grocery shopping spree. Doing so helps keep perishable foods safe to eat, because you'll want to get them home and in the fridge as soon as possible.

>> **Keep produce on the top.** Place fruits and vegetables in plastic bags to keep them safe for consumption. To maintain the freshness of produce or eggs, avoid placing heavy items on top of them.

>> **Sort foods when placing on conveyor belt.** When checking out and placing your items on the belt, try to arrange them by food groups to make it faster for you to unload/organize at home. Ask the bagger to keep fresh meats/poultry in separate bags away from fresh produce (safer) and keep cold/frozen items together (to help keep them cold). If using self-checkout, follow the same bagging routine.

Favoring farmers' markets

Heading to farmers' markets compared to grocery stores has a couple benefits. The food at farmers' markets is fresher, seasonal, locally grown (you support local farmers), and you get a better variety of foods. Frequenting your local farmers' market is the ultimate health food store!

The following foods are some of the best to buy at your local farmers' market:

>> **Tomatoes:** Buy vine ripened and store with stem up. Green at the top is perfectly fine because tomatoes continue to ripen — just be sure to avoid storing in the refrigerator, which will surely rob the tomatoes of their flavor.

>> **Peaches, apricots, and nectarines:** They continue to ripen so buy them according to when you think you'll eat them. Immediately eat a sweet, fully ripened spectacularly delicious farm-fresh peach.

>> **Cantaloupe:** Let your nose do the picking. A ripe cantaloupe has a sweet melon smell at the stem end.

>> **Berries:** Berries don't ripen after picking so buy the ones that look full and plump and ready to pop in your mouth at the market. A strawberry, for example, should be red and ripe all the way to the top. Just be sure not to wash the berries until right before you're ready to eat them.

>> **Cucumbers:** Look for green and firm cucumbers, never yellow, which is an indication of aging.

>> **Eggplants:** Focus on shiny, smooth, deeply colored eggplants — never wrinkled, which indicates aging.

>> **Lettuce:** Look at the stem of the lettuce: If it is brown, it's a sure indication the head isn't fresh. Also, look for lettuce that still contains much of the outer leaves. Sellers remove outer leaves to mask signs of aging. If buying bin lettuce, look for fresh-looking leaves that aren't brown in color or wilted.

>> **Corn:** Check the stem of the corn stalk; brown stems indicate aging. Also, break off part of the stalk to inspect the kernels. Look for wrinkled or wilted looking kernels which again indicates the cob is not fresh.

>> **Avocados:** To ensure your avocado is ripe, inspect the cap. If the avocado is unripe, the cap can't be removed. If you pop off the cap and it is brown under the cap, the avocado is overripe. Green under the cap is just right. A slightly soft (but not mushy) feel is another indication of ripeness.

TIP

Buy organic produce when available. Refer to the section, "Going organic," later in this chapter.

Knowing How to Read Labels

Packaged foods have nutrition labels on them called Nutrition Facts. These numbers give you valuable information about the nutritional quality of the food you're buying. When you're following an intermittent fasting plan, discover how to read a Nutrition Facts label, and you can easily boost your nutrition and make healthier choices.

The FDA has given a facelift to the old Nutrition Facts label. The new label will be required on all packaged foods made in the United States and imported from other countries. The new label is slated to appear on most packages by January 1, 2021. Figure 18-2 is a label; refer to it as you read the following bulleted list.

TIP

For a quick scan technique, pick up the food product and pay attention to the crucial information that will help you to decide then and there whether to put the food back on the shelf or in your cart. Here's what to look for:

>> **Serving size:** Look to see how many servings the package contains. Servings can be the most deceiving number of all the numbers on the label. How many times do you zero in on the calories and assume that low number is for the entire package? Compare serving sizes among products. Check how many servings you're eating. (Odds are you're eating more than you think.) Figure 18-2 shows a product with a ⅔ of a cup serving size, but there are 8 servings per container!

Nutrition Facts

8 servings per container
Serving size   2/3 cup (55g)

Amount per serving
Calories   230

	% Daily Value*
Total Fat 8g	**10%**
Saturated Fat 1g	**5%**
Trans Fat 0g	
Cholesterol 0mg	**0%**
Sodium 160mg	**7%**
Total Carbohydrate 37g	**13%**
Dietary Fiber 4g	**14%**
Total Sugars 12g	
Includes 10g Added Sugars	**20%**
Protein 3g	
Vitamin D 2mcg	10%
Calcium 260mg	20%
Iron 8mg	45%
Potassium 240mg	6%

* The % Daily Value (DV) tells you how much a nutrient in a serving of food contributes to a daily diet. 2,000 calories a day is used for general nutrition advice.

FIGURE 18-2:
A sample Nutrition Facts label.

Source: www.fda.gov

>> **Calories:** Identify how many calories you'll be eating in each serving. Don't forget, if the package contains four servings, then multiply the calories time four! This product contains 230 calories per serving, but if you ate the entire container, you'd be eating 1,840 calories.

>> **Total fat, saturated fat, and trans fat:** Zero in on the saturated fat. Make sure to choose products where the percentage Daily Value of saturated fat is under 5 percent. If the food has any trans fat whatsoever, put it back. Figure 18-2 shows an acceptable food, with just 1 gram of saturated fat and 0 gram trans fat.

>> **Cholesterol:** Only animal foods contain cholesterol. Make sure to choose products where the percentage Daily Value of cholesterol is under 5 percent. Figure 18-2 shows a 0mg cholesterol food — always a good sign.

>> **Sodium:** The food supply has far too much sodium for promoting good health. Choose foods with the lowest sodium count (make sure to choose products where the percentage Daily Value of sodium is under 5 percent). Figure 18-2 has too much sodium (more than 5 percent Daily Value per serving).

TIP

>> **Dietary fiber:** Check to see whether the product is high in healthy fiber. Look for products with a percent Daily Value of 20 percent or more. Less than 5 percent is low, so put it back. Figure 18-2 has more than 5 percent Daily Value, so it's a higher fiber food.

Health organizations suggest a daily intake of 25 grams of dietary fiber for women and 38 grams for men to protect against disease. However, the average American eats only about half that much (about 15 grams per day). One easy way to bump up your daily fiber intake is to choose whole grains over refined (think brown). Buy breads with at least 3 grams of fiber per serving and whole grains as the first ingredient.

>> **Total Sugars:** Too much sugar adds weight and promotes cardiovascular disease. Look to see whether the product is loaded with sugar. Look for products with less than 3 grams of "Total Sugars." Figure 18-2 has far too much sugar (12 grams), 20 percent Daily Value, which is too high.

>> **Vitamins and minerals:** Check for products with 20 percent or more of at least one of the vitamins or minerals listed. Figure 18-2 has a good amount of calcium and iron.

Flip to the front of the product and you may see a nutrition claim used by manufacturers to draw consumers' attention. You'll see numerous *nutrition claims*, all with specific meaning such as if the label reads "Fat free," which means that a single serving has less than 0.5g fat. Here is general guidance on what the claims mean:

>> *Free* means a food has the least possible amount of the specified nutrient.

>> *Very low* and *low* means the food has a little more than foods labeled *free.*

>> *Reduced* or *less* mean the food has 25 percent less of a specific nutrient than the regular product.

>> *More, fortified, enriched, added, extra,* or *plus* means the food has 10 percent or more of the Daily Value (DV) than the regular product. They may only be used for vitamins, minerals, protein, dietary fiber, and potassium.

WARNING

Watch out for misleading claims. Misdirected health claims are misguided statements made by producers that lead consumers to believe a food is healthier than it actually is. Examples include foods that are labeled "low in fat" or "low in carbohydrates," yet still high in calories. A food package claim on a box of cookies, may read something like "high in calcium" or "no high fructose corn syrup" to make you think the product is healthy, when in fact those cookies are loaded with cane sugar and calories and have no fiber.

Sizing up the ingredient list

The ingredients list is one of the easiest ways to size up if a food is healthy or not. All foods must list the ingredients in *descending order* of predominance by weight. That means the ingredients with the largest amounts in the product are listed first, and the ones with the smallest amounts are at the end of the list. This concept is important for checking the proportion of sugar or sodium added to the product. Follow these guidelines for interpreting the ingredients on the label:

For example, compare the ingredients list of two boxes of popular cereals:

>> **Cereal #1:** Whole grain oats, corn starch, sugar, salt, tripotassium phosphate. vitamin E (mixed tocopherols) added to preserve freshness. vitamins and minerals: calcium carbonate, iron and zinc (mineral nutrients), vitamin C (sodium ascorbate), a B vitamin (niacinamide), vitamin B6 (pyridoxine hydrochloride), vitamin A (palmitate), vitamin B, (thiamin mononitrate), a B vitamin (folic acid), vitamin B12, vitamin D3.

>> **Cereal #2:** Sugar, Wheat, Corn Syrup, Honey, Hydrogenated Soybean Oil (Less than 0.5g Trans Fat per Serving), Salt, Caramel Color, Soy Lecithin. Vitamins: Sodium Ascorbate (vitamin C), Niacinamide, Pyridoxine Hydrochloride (vitamin B6), Riboflavin (vitamin B2), Thiamin Hydrochloride (vitamin B1), vitamin A palmitate, Folic Acid, vitamin B12 and vitamin D. To Maintain Quality, BHT Has Been Added to the Packaging.

Notice that the first ingredient in Cereal #1 is whole grain oats, whereas the first ingredient in the Cereal #2 is sugar. Cereal #2 has double the sugar (18 grams) per serving compared to Cereal #1 (9 grams of sugar per serving).

Hydrogenated soybean oil is an indication that Cereal #2 contain trans fat. *Trans fat* is created when food manufacturers take a liquid polyunsaturated vegetable oil and turn it into a solid fat by a chemical process called *hydrogenation*. Trans fats, even if consumed in small portions, fuels the progression of heart disease. It's never safe to eat any trans fats, so stay away at all cost! The best way to tell if a food contains trans fat is to look on the labels for trans fat content or an easier way is simply to scan the ingredients list for the word hydrogenated. If it says "hydrogenated," put the product back on the shelf.

Searching for sugar

Added sugar — sugar that isn't naturally a part of the food you eat — is where the problem lies. Note that the new labels were changed to include the amount of added sugar the food contains. The United States' sugar addiction has been linked to numerous health concerns such as obesity, metabolic syndrome, and insulin resistance. In fact, the average adult American eats a whopping 22 teaspoons of added sugar a day, mostly from liquid sugar, also known as soda and other processed, sweetened foods. That's four times more than what the American Heart Association recommends people restrict their daily added sugar intake to for better health: *no more than 5 to 9 teaspoons* (20 to 36 grams) of added sugar per day. Take the first step in curbing your sweet tooth: Cut way back on soda and sugary snacks and eat more of Mother Nature's naturally sweet treats — fresh fruit.

If you have a sweet tooth, incorporate these tricks I use to limit added sugars and make sure you don't blow your overall daily calorie budget:

>> **Eat natural, whole foods, like fruits, vegetables, nuts, and seeds, because added sugars are primarily in processed foods.** This is especially true for snacks, because between-meal noshes are often sugar-laden.

>> **Avoid processed food as much as possible.** As a general rule, the more processed a food is, the higher percentage of its sugars are added.

>> **Check the ingredient list.** For a better idea of the added sugar content, look at the ingredient list on packaged foods. If any of these terms are among the first three ingredients, the food is sugar-rich: brown sugar, corn sweetener, corn syrup, sugar (dextrose, fructose, glucose, sucrose), high-fructose corn syrup, honey, invert sugar, malt sugar, molasses, raw sugar, or syrup.

>> **Choose foods labeled low-sugar, sugar-free, or sugar-reduced.** An easy way to ensure the food is low in added sugars is to check the front of the box for one of the *nutrition claims*.

>> **Pay particular attention to common sugar culprits.** These foods and beverages listed here are guiltiest because they're the most common sources of added sugars in the diet:

- Regular soft drinks: 33 percent contribution to total added sugar intake
- Straight sugar and candy: 16 percent
- Cakes, cookies, pies: 13 percent
- Fruit drinks and "-ades" (not 100 percent fruit juice): 10 percent
- Dairy (watch out for sweetened yogurt and ice cream): 8.5 percent
- Grain-based foods (watch out for cinnamon toast and sweetened cereals): 6 percent

Added sugars may be disguised in the Nutrition Facts label under the following words: corn sugar, corn syrup, high-fructose corn syrup, invert sugar, honey, glucose, dextrin, brown sugar, maple, dextrose, fructose, maltose, and levulose.

Slashing the sodium

The food supply is tainted. The fact is that salt, a prized condiment, is actually a slow poison. Excess sodium intake is inextricably linked to the development of serious diseases in both women and men, namely heart disease (the No. 1 killer) and stroke (the No. 3 killer). In fact, a whopping 90 percent of people will eventually develop high blood pressure from a lifetime of too much salt. The words *salt* and *sodium* are sometimes used interchangeably because most of the sodium people eat is in the form of salt. Think of salt as the transport vehicle for the dangerous mineral, sodium. Sodium is a mineral that is harmful.

The American Heart Association recommends no more than 2,300 milligrams (mg) of sodium a day and moving toward an ideal limit of no more than 1,500 mg of sodium per day (3.8 grams of salt) for most adults. Americans consume almost three times that amount or about 4,000 milligrams of sodium or 10 grams salt, per day. (One quarter of adult men get more than 5,200 mg per day, and one quarter of adult women consume more than 3,500 mg per day.) That's the major reason why nearly half of adults in the United States (108 million, or 45 percent) have high blood pressure (also known as the silent killer).

TIP

Keep your arteries healthy and your blood pressure down by consuming no more than 2,400 milligrams of sodium per day (about 1 teaspoon salt), and even less (1,500 milligrams) if you're middle-aged or older and/or have high blood pressure.

Sodium is often hidden in food products, so make sure you become a food label sleuth. Pay particular attention to processed foods. As you scrutinize the ingredients list, watch out for the trilogy of "S" words: *salt, sodium, and soda* as well as the chemical nomenclature *Na*. Beware of these words:

Monosodium glutamate (MSG)

Baking powder

Sodium alginate

Sodium ascorbate

Sodium bicarbonate (baking soda)

Sodium benzoate

Sodium chloride

Sodium caseinate

Sodium citrate

Sodium hydroxide

Sodium nitrate

Sodium saccharin

Sodium stearoyl lactylate

Sodium sulfite

Disodium phosphate

Trisodium phosphate

About 75 percent of a person's total salt intake comes from salt added to processed foods by manufacturers and salt that cooks add to foods at restaurants and other food service establishments. So, if your food comes primarily in a box, a bag, a can, or off a menu, the odds are it's too high in sodium.

REMEMBER

The best way to keep your sodium intake in check is to cook at home and use fresh whole foods seasoned with herbs, spices, citrus, vinegars, and EVOO and use salt sparingly in the kitchen. Cut back on your intake of processed foods (bagged, boxed, and canned). If you're buying processed foods, choose foods with a value of *less than 20* on the % Daily Value from sodium. The average American eats approximately 10 grams of salt a day, which is far more than the 5 to 6 grams health professionals recommend. Cutting salt by a mere 3 grams a day (about 400 mg sodium) would mean 6 percent fewer new cases of heart disease, 8 percent fewer heart attacks, and 3 percent fewer deaths.

Rating the frozen meals

Stroll down any supermarket frozen food aisle and the evidence is clear: Frozen meals are wildly popular, claiming more shelf space than virtually any other type of frozen food. There are easy ways to bypass the crowd and zero in on the healthiest frozen foods.

TIP

Try to add a side salad and a serving of fruit to round out your frozen meal, especially if you're having a lower-calorie frozen dinner. Not only will it boost the vitamin, mineral, and fiber content, but the extra fruit and vegetables will help fill you up.

When perusing the frozen food aisle, look for plant-based meals. As a general rule, focus on entrees that include plenty of vegetables. They tend to be lower in calories and higher in vitamins and minerals as well as fiber (which also helps fill you up). Look for brown rice or whole grains whenever possible, and choose bean, fish, or chicken entrees. Check the stats on the package nutrition label and follow these guidelines:

By the numbers, here are guidelines for choosing a healthier frozen meal:

1. **Look for frozen meals labeled as *light*.**

   The FDA defines *light* as a food that has been significantly reduced in fat, calories, or sodium.

2. **Choose meals low in saturated fat.**

   Aim for less than 4 grams.

3. **Choose meals with a maximum of 800 milligrams of sodium.**

   Lower is better.

4. **Select meals with a minimum of 3 to 5 grams of fiber.**

WARNING

Most frozen dinners are loaded with fat, sodium, and calories, so be sure to check the serving size. Look to see whether the nutrition facts are for the entire package or a portion. Read the label and choose wisely!

For example, a quick and easy frozen food meal would be a frozen cheddar cheese, bean, and rice burrito, light in sodium. Pair it with a fresh arugula salad dressed simply with extra virgin olive oil and a squeeze of fresh lemon juice, and you have a healthy meal or snack in minutes.

Going organic

If you're concerned about pesticides and herbicides and prefer to buy organically grown food, look for products that contain the USDA organic symbol. USDA certified organic foods are grown and processed according to federal guidelines addressing, among many factors, soil quality, animal-raising practices, pest and weed control, and the use of additives. Organic producers rely on natural substances and physical, mechanical, or biologically based farming methods to the fullest extent possible.

WEB EXTRAS

Produce doesn't contain the USDA certification. The Environmental Working Group is a nonprofit activist group (www.ewg.org/) that specializes in research and advocacy in the areas of agricultural subsidies, toxic chemicals, drinking water pollutants, and corporate accountability. Every year the group releases two lists: the "dirty dozen" and the "clean 15." These lists can help you to decide which produce you should buy that is organically grown and which conventional produce is perfectly fine to buy. Here is the 2020 dirty dozen foods list in descending order:

- >> Strawberries
- >> Spinach
- >> Kale
- >> Nectarines
- >> Apples
- >> Grapes
- >> Peaches
- >> Cherries
- >> Pears
- >> Tomatoes
- >> Celery
- >> Potatoes

Chapter **19**

Stocking Your Fridge, Freezer, and Pantry with Nutrition

t's five o'clock: Your eating window is starting, and you're really hungry. What's for dinner? Tired from a long day and unwilling to spend an hour in the kitchen or even order in, you wonder what exactly your options are for a quick and healthy dinner. The best way to prepare for this inevitable scenario is to have a stocked and organized healthy pantry and refrigerator.

Unfortunately, many people report that a shortage of time is the greatest challenge to getting in the kitchen and cooking healthy, delicious meals. This chapter explains why keeping well-planned food supplies is the best way to ensure you'll get healthy meals at home on days you just don't feel like spending a long period of time cooking.

Cooking meals from scratch is one of the most important actions you can take for your health over your lifetime. This chapter shows you how to simplify your life and save oodles of time in the kitchen. If you're organized and prepared, you can get a healthy and delicious meal on the table in less than the time it takes to order and pickup takeout.

Organizing a Healthy Refrigerator

Every refrigerator has a general internal layout. Separate spaces are designed for storing dairy, meat, cheeses, beverages, eggs, leftovers, and dressings — all separated from each other. Knowing the correct space to put your food items is step one in your kitchen makeover. The following sections help plot out the spaces in your fridge and freezer so you can maximize the space you have and be successful on your intermittent fasting plan.

Putting things in place

You may be surprised to know that refrigerator manufacturers assume you know the laws of what goes where in a refrigerator, yet few people read the instructions. Every refrigerator has top, middle, and lower shelves and door storage. Here are suggestions for placing your perishables in the safest places:

>> **Top shelves:** Keep low-fat or skim milk and/or nondairy milks and yogurts (preferably fat-free) on the higher shelves, toward the back (the coldest spots), and not on the door. Keep leftovers in clear containers, at your eye level, and eat them soon. Position some ready-to-eat fruits and veggies for quick snacks at the front and center of your refrigerator. Store them on the first shelf, nearest eye level. This way, you can reach them easily when you're hungry or when looking for something to eat (during your eating windows).

FOOD SAFETY REFRIGERATOR BASICS

Here are some reminders to ensure your food is safe. Making sure you avoid nasty bacterial infections that can spoil your food is important:

- Keep the temperature at no greater than 40° F and no less than 32° F.

- Always cover food and don't overload the refrigerator; food should have room for air to circulate and keep it cool.

- Cool hot foods in the refrigerator (separate them into smaller containers first) and make sure to defrost foods and marinate food in the fridge, never on the counter.

- Leave the open bottles/containers in the front, so you can use them first.

- Double wrap raw fish/poultry and isolate in the refrigerator to prevent cross-contamination of bacteria onto other foods.

>> **Middle and lower shelves:** Store eggs in their original cardboard crates on a shelf and not on the refrigerator door. Store egg substitutes or egg white liquid cartons on the colder top shelf with the dairy. If your fridge doesn't have a drawer for cheeses, take a small clear container and organize all the cheeses into the container. Choose low fat/fat-free versions such as unrefrigerated creamy cheese wedges, farmer's cheese, cottage cheese, and mozzarella. Try flavoring your food with a small amount of strong cheese such as Parmesan, Romano, or asiago, shredded. Take another small clear container and place the fish, seafood, and poultry next to the cheese container (make sure you eat these foods within a day or so or else freeze them).

>> **Crisper drawers:** Keep fragile fruits and vegetables stored in the appropriate crisper drawers at the bottom of your fridge. As a general rule, use the low humidity setting for anything that rots easily, such as apples, pears, avocados, melons, or stone fruits. The high humidity drawer is for anything that wilts — think thin-skinned vegetables like asparagus or leafy greens and fresh herbs. If your fridge doesn't have a drawer for fruits, take a small clear container and organize all the fruits into the container. You may also consider buying protective produce drawer liners to keep your fruit and vegetables fresh longer.

>> **Fridge door:** Keep the most frequently used beverages in the fridge door and group the remaining least-used on the top and back of the tallest shelf. Keep water and low-sodium vegetable juices handy. Dressings and condiments should also go in the door. Keep the most-used condiments in the front of the fridge door and group the remaining dressings and sauces toward the back of the shortest shelf. Have the reduced-fat versions of dressings and other healthy condiments available, including horseradish, salsa, mustards, relish, and low-sodium and low-sugar ketchup. More healthy condiment ideas include pesto, minced or whole peeled garlic, hummus, roasted red peppers, and sun-dried tomatoes.

Establishing a well-stocked freezer

Your freezer needs to be organized and well-stocked. Whether you have a side-by-side freezer, drawer freezer, or even a deep freeze chest, staying organized is the key to quick and healthy meals. Here are some freezer organizational tips:

>> **Use clear plastic bins.** To help you organize your freezer foods, use inexpensive plastic bins. Label them to give you individual spaces for all the foods you store.

>> **Remove from boxes.** Oftentimes the foods in the frozen section come in large bulky boxes. If possible, save space by removing food from boxes and store in containers.

>> **Freeze things flat.** If possible, place foods such as leftovers in a freezer bag. Use a food sealer to tightly seal your bags and remove all the air. After your freezer bags are frozen, you can stand them up on their sides because they're only about an inch wide.

>> **Label everything.** To help you keep track of what food you have and when it needs to be used by, be sure to write the name and date on the food.

Every healthy Mediterranean-style freezer has five general categories of foods:

>> **Lean proteins:** Use one section of your freezer for protein. Keep pre-portioned servings of frozen fish fillets such as wild salmon fillets, tuna steaks, shrimp, and scallops. Keep a supply of meatless burger patties for a super-fast burger dinner. Pre-portioned skinless chicken breasts should also be handy.

>> **Breads:** Another section of your freezer should be for grain products. Keep 100 percent whole grain breads, pizza dough, waffles, English muffins, and other grains handy for last-minute meals.

>> **Frozen desserts:** Another bin can be used for frozen desserts. Include frozen fruit bars, fat-free ice cream, and frozen yogurt.

>> **Frozen fruits and vegetables:** Use another bin for fruits and veggies. Keep frozen fruit (without added sugar) for smoothies and baking. Frozen veggies (ensure your frozen vegetables are plain, 100 percent vegetables, meaning they should be the only things on the ingredient list) also come in handy for quick stir-fries.

>> **Ready-to-eat meals:** Have a section of complete, healthy frozen meals. For those days when cooking just isn't in the cards, have some quick and healthy frozen meals ready to pop in the microwave. Flip to Chapter 18 for a guide to choosing the healthiest frozen food meals.

Arranging a Healthy Pantry

One major step in creating an organized kitchen is to make your pantry a lean, mean, fighting machine. To do so, ensure you have an organized and well-stocked pantry, filled with all the things you need to create healthful meals, lickety-split.

TIP

Junk food is loaded with calories, salt, sugar, and/or bad fats. Because the food contains unhealthy ingredients and is low in nutrition, nutritionists refer to this type of food as *empty calorie foods* to reflect their lack of nutrients. In order to kick the junk food habit, don't have it around in the first place to tempt you is the best advice. Don't buy it, even when you find a great sale. To create a pantry suitable to an intermittent faster, throw out the junk food immediately and replace it with healthier foods. Remember to choose your calories by the nutrient companions they keep and in so doing, get the biggest bang for your calorie bite. Chapter 18 helps you decipher labels.

Organizing your pantry will take some thought and time in the beginning, but your efforts will surely pay off with by saving you time and money in the future.

Capitalizing on categories

Figuring out a system for storing your pantry items is a life hack that will make your life easier and cut a huge chunk of time out of your meal prep. Having an organized pantry and your home food supplies can make an enormous difference when you're following an intermittent fast and eating healthier. Follow these tips to organize your pantry with healthful food choices that will make your new healthy eating lifestyle a breeze:

1. **Take everything out of the cupboards for starters.**

   Clean the shelves before putting the stuff back.

2. **Organize with bins and containers.**

   Reorganize using containers you can find at the dollar store, so you can pull foods out of the pantry easily. Group them by type, most used, or whatever makes sense for your family. Refer to the next section for more tips about how you can organize the items.

3. **Check the dates.**

   Get rid of anything that is years past the expiration date or if the can has dents in it. That said, many foods are completely safe to eat, even past the expiration date.

WEB EXTRAS

   If you're not sure whether a product or item is worth saving past its date label, a free app called FoodKeeper, created by the USDA's Food Safety and Inspection Service with Cornell University and the Food Marketing Institute (www.foodsafety.gov/keep-food-safe/foodkeeper-app) will help.

4. **Restock by category, starting with the oldest date first.**

   Put back only the items you use. Organize things in a way that works for you: all canned goods together, nut butters together, cereal, and so on. You can even consider doing it alphabetically.

TIP

   Always keep some healthy choices front and center. Keep your less healthful foods in hard-to-reach places — places like way at the bottom of the pantry, in the back, or way up top.

Knowing what and where to store food

Try stocking up on these easy-to-prepare, yet healthy, staples in your home pantry:

» **Grains:** Take a small clear plastic bin and label it "Grains." Add your boxes of grains into the bin. Think shades of brown (and orange) for healthy whole grains, such as rolled and/or steel-cut oats, barley, brown rice, wild rice, and popcorn, and the more exotic types, such as quinoa, bulgur, amaranth, wheat berries, and millet. Next to the grain bin, put your boxes of ready-to-eat whole grain cereal.

» **Beans:** For your bean shelf, label a small clear plastic container "Beans." Put in all your packaged legumes, which are fiber-rich and antioxidant-packed lean sources of protein, such as packets of dried beans, lentils (great for adding fiber and protein to pasta; check out the Lentil Soup recipe in Chapter 21), and peas (check out the Split Pea Soup recipe in Chapter 21). Place the canned beans (preferably low or no sodium) like chickpeas for salads and black beans, together on the shelf next to the container.

» **Pasta and tomatoes:** Put all pasta in a small, labeled container "Pasta." Add boxes of whole grain pasta. Try some of the other healthy pastas such as quinoa, chickpea, buckwheat, and brown rice varieties. On the shelf next to the container, put your bottles of tomato sauce (watch the sodium count on the sauces). Add cans of tomato products (preferably low or no sodium) like diced tomatoes and tomato paste.

» **Fruits and vegetables:** Another shelf can be for your "Fruits/Veggies." Add cans of fruit (in natural juices), containers of 100 percent fruit juice, and cans of vegetables and vegetable soups (preferably low in sodium).

» **Nuts and seeds:** Grab another small clear container and label it "Nuts." Add bags/cans of unsalted natural walnuts, pistachios, and almonds. Don't forget the no-salt-added nut butters. You can also put tahini here. Add chia seeds, pumpkin seeds, sunflower seeds, and sealed packets of ground flaxseed (flaxseeds must be ground before eating). Open bags of ground flaxseeds are highly perishable and must be stored in a sealed container and refrigerated.

» **Canned fish:** Label another small clear container "Fish." Add water-packed cans or packs of tuna and salmon, plus cans of clams and other favorite fish products.

» **Broths:** In another clear container or section of your pantry is where you consolidate your "Broths." Add cans of reduced sodium broths (chicken, beef, vegetable) for steaming vegetables, flavoring soups, and other healthy cooking techniques.

>> **Dried herbs and spice bottles:** To organize them, buy a three-tiered, expandable, adjustable pantry organizer and arrange your spice and herb bottles in alphabetical order. Getting organized means your spices and herbs will always be at the ready and that you'll be able to keep track of what you have and won't buy spices and herbs that you already have.

TIP

Whole spices will stay fresh for about 4 years, ground spices for about 2 to 3 years and dried herbs for 1 to 3 years. Store spices in a cool, dark cupboard, away from direct heat or sunlight; keep tightly closed when not in use.

>> **Condiments:** Take another small clear container and label it "Condiments" or use a designated section in your pantry. Add all sorts of healthy condiments such as mustards, vinegars, and hot sauce to add flavor to your food without added salt. Be sure to refrigerate opened condiments that have a "refrigerate after opening" statement on the label. In general, fermented sauces (soy, Worcestershire), hot sauces, nut butters, and honey can be left out. Refer to the nearby sidebar for a list of healthful condiments.

>> **Baking supplies:** Label another small clear container "Baking." Add baking necessities such as baking soda, baking powder, muffin cups, vanilla extract, dark chocolate chips, dark chocolate cocoa powder, sugar, sugar substitutes, and flour. You can also add nonfat dry milk and cans of fat-free condensed milk to this container. Refined flour lasts up to one year whereas you can expect a shelf life of only one to three months for whole grain flour stored at cool room temperature. For longer storage, stash your flour in the freezer.

>> **Oils and vinegars:** Clear an area of your pantry shelf for healthy oils such as extra virgin olive oil (EVOO), canola, flaxseed, and an array of cooking sprays. Add an assortment of fine vinegars (well-aged balsamic and balsamic glaze) regular vinegars like white, rice and cider, dry sherry, and wine for cooking (albeit it's best to use a chardonnay or cabernet for your cooking wine needs).

>> **Snacks:** Another area of your pantry is for snacks. These include popcorn kernels, whole grain crackers, unsweetened apple sauce, fruit leather, dried fruits (apricots, dates, and raisins), baked chips, rice cakes, and shelf-stable fat-free pudding cups.

>> **Extra plant-based milks:** A small area of your pantry can be for shelf-stable milks, including boxed unsweetened plain soymilk or unsweetened plain almond milk.

TIP

If pantry space is limited, and you don't have room for all the containers, buy a three-tier riser that will fit on a pantry shelf. Using a riser in a pantry enables you to store a bunch of items in one spot while allowing you to see everything you have at once.

CONDIMENTS TO FLAVOR YOUR FOOD AND YOUR LIFE

If you're tired of the same old fish dinner, try adding some zip to your zucchini and flavor to your fish with some of my favorite condiments:

- Balsamic vinegar

- Chili powder

- Dijon mustard

- Harissa

- Honey mustard

- Horseradish

- Hot sauce

- Pesto

- Salsa

- Wasabi

REMEMBER

Having a well-stocked kitchen translates into being able to whip up a healthy meal in minutes. For example, here's a quick and healthy dinner idea: Boil up some whole wheat pasta; drain, and place in a serving bowl. Heat your favorite bottled tomato sauce (preferably low in sodium) and pour over the pasta. Top with shavings of a strong and flavorful cheese such as Parmigiano-Reggiano. Serve with a veggie-packed salad — with added beans (rinsed of excess sodium). Dress the salad with EVOO, flavored vinegar, and a spritz of fresh lemon juice, and you have an ultra-fast and healthy dinner in minutes, plus you'll have a complete protein that increases your fiber and antioxidant intake.

Chapter **20**

Making Cooking at Home a Delicious Habit

ood health begins at home. The fact is, when you eat at home, you eat healthier and lighter. That's because *you* have control of the ingredients as well as the portion size. In general, meals prepared outside the home are higher in calories and less healthy than foods prepared at home. When dining out, people tend to eat larger portions, loaded with excess calories, fat, and salt.

So, before you enjoy making healthy eating at home a way of life, make sure you have a well-stocked kitchen. Having kitchen essentials on hand is the key to simplifying the process of cooking, meal-prepping, and creating healthy and delicious food for you and your family. In this chapter, I explain how you can make your *home where the health is,* including advice about stocking your kitchen and cooking healthy.

A well-stocked kitchen is key for creating sustainable, nutritious eating habits. Having the most essential cooking tools at your fingertips will make your life so much easier. Although the culinary world frequently touts sleek, trendy, and exciting new kitchen gadgets all the time, you don't need to buy them to be able to cook well. In fact, the most basic tools are all you need to start cooking delicious meals.

Simplifying Your Cooking and Your Life

One of the main goals of intermittent fasting is to simplify your life, which includes eating and cooking fewer meals and less cleaning up afterward. Simplifying your life will give you more time, space, and energy. The more space you have, the freer you'll be to truly enjoy everything. A functional, efficient, organized, and clutter-free kitchen saves you time, energy, money and stress.

Whether you're a hesitant beginner or an expert cook, everyone who sets foot in a kitchen sometimes needs a refresher on the basics. The following sections look at the fundamental culinary tools that will make your cooking experience easier, although don't feel it's necessary to run out and buy everything right now to make your intermittent fasting program successful. This is a dream list; you can build it up over time.

Cookware

Here is a list of standard cookware that you may already have in your kitchen. If not, consider adding them to your kitchen:

>> **A cast iron skillet:** Cast iron skillets have been used for hundreds of years to sear, sauté, and roast an array of food items — a true kitchen workhorse. Although the inexpensive and highly versatile skillet is a chef's favorite, many people worry about the potential for iron overload. Cast iron cookware is a potential source of iron in your diet — this may be viewed as one of the advantages or disadvantages of using cast iron cookware. Iron (an essential mineral) does leach into food, especially when considering the type of food being cooked (moisture and acidity) as well as the length of cooking time. Many groups benefit from getting more iron in their diet, including women and children. But too much iron in the diet isn't good for everyone, such as those individuals with *hemochromatosis* (a genetic disorder where too much iron builds up in your body).

TIP

Properly seasoning your cast iron cookware prevents it from rusting. To season your skillet, coat the entire skillet (inside and out) with olive oil and bake in the oven at 400° Fahrenheit for an hour.

>> **A stainless-steel cookware set:** If you can afford to invest in a professional grade cookware set, go for it. The versatility and durability are well worth the money because they'll last a lifetime.

>> **A nonstick frying pan:** Every household needs at least one super versatile pan to sauté vegetables, make sauces, and whip up pancakes. Just be careful to use nonabrasive tools to avoid damaging the surface.

>> **A glass baking dish:** A microwave-safe 8-inch glass baking dish is perfect for casseroles and even brownies. For dishes made with acidic ingredients such as tomatoes and lemon, always bake in glass because other types of metal dishes can react with these foods and cause the foods to discolor. Even more convenient, the small size of this dish can fit in the microwave to save you time. Remember to never broil food in a glass dish because the high temperatures may cause the glass to shatter.

>> **Baking sheets:** A couple of rimmed baking sheets are indispensable kitchen tools that you may not have considered including in your kitchen. A rimmed baking sheet is thin, lightweight, and much easier to store than a roasting pan. For example, if you're roasting broccoli florets or a whole fish, this should be your pan of choice.

A silicone baking mat for lining your sheet is also a fabulous cooking tool. The mat is an endless reusable alternative to foil that you do *not* have to liberally spray. Just a tiny spritz of nonstick spray, and nothing ever burns, sticks, or peels. Trust me, these pans can get a lot of action, including roasting vegetables, toasting nuts, and of course, baking cookies.

Utensils

This section looks at another category of kitchen essentials — utensils — that will significantly ease your meal prep routines:

>> **A great set of knives:** Perhaps nothing simplifies your kitchen experience more than great cutting knives. A trusty set of top rated knifes can do it all — slicing, mincing, dicing, and chopping. If an entire set isn't in your budget, invest in one or two razor sharp and incredibly versatile chef's knives. You may also consider a knife sharpener, which is a great addition to keep your knives super sharp.

>> **Stainless measuring spoons:** A set of durable stainless-steel measuring spoons is a requirement for precisely adding dry ingredients during food prep and cooking. The strong stainless-steel construction will last forever.

>> **Glass measuring cups:** Generations of cooks have relied on durable glass measuring cups. Marked in red for at-a-glance precision, this high-quality tempered glass can safely be used in the dishwasher, freezer, fridge, microwave, and oven.

>> **A sharp peeler:** Investing in a sharp vegetable peeler will not only save you time but also save you a lot of aggravation in the kitchen. Although a vegetable peeler may seem like a humble tool, it's a crucially important one. A sharp blade, comfortable grip, and smooth movements can make the difference

between hacking away at your potatoes and having an effortless peeling experience. Use it to peel your vegetables and shave cheese or make veggie ribbons. My favorite are the Swiss-made peelers with a carbon steel blade that starts and stays sharper.

>> **A whisk:** A whisk is a must-have tool for emulsifying oil and vinegar dressings and marinades.

>> **Tongs:** Tongs are extremely useful for moving around large pieces of food and flipping hot foods on a baking sheet without the risk of burns.

Tools and gadgets

There is a whole world of enticing kitchen gadgets to choose from, and it can be hard to know what's really worth your time and money. Here is a list of tools and gadgets that will really make a difference in the amount of time it takes you to prep and cook, how well things turn out, and how fast cleanup goes afterward:

>> **A food processor:** Nothing comes in handier than this incredibly versatile kitchen gadget. For example, you can easily whip up homemade pesto, salsa, breadcrumbs, nut butters, puréed vegetables, soups, and hummus with the touch of a button. You can use it to chop vegetables, herbs, seeds, and hard cheeses.

>> **Wood cutting boards:** The best cutting board material is one that can be easily cleaned and doesn't damage or dull knives. Wood is still the best choice. Have two:

- One strictly to cut raw meat, poultry, and seafood

- Another to cut ready-to-eat foods, like breads and vegetables

After each use and before moving on to the next step while prepping food, clean the cutting boards thoroughly in hot, soapy water, and then rinse them with water and air dry or pat dry with clean paper towels.

>> **Instant read thermometer:** Using an instant-read thermometer will make sure your meals are *always* perfectly done. Because the animal proteins you'll be eating are mostly fish and skinless poultry, remember these temperatures to ensure that the heat has killed off any potentially harmful germs and protects you and your family from food-borne illnesses.

- **Fish:** 160° F

- **Chicken and other poultry:** 165°F

» **A blender:** Nothing says smoothie better than a blender. When differentiating between an old-fashioned blender, a juicer, and the newer super-fast versions, it's all in the design of the blades. A blender and the fast style mixers are better than juicers, because you mix up the entire food, whereas a juicer loses much of the healthy fiber. The difference between an old-fashioned blender and the new super-fast blenders is that the cyclonic action and higher RPM of the fast blender creates a significantly more appetizing drink than older blenders, which simply can't break down harder foods to the same degree. If buying a super-fast style blender, choose the most powerful version, the one with a 700-watt motor.

» **Stainless set of nonskid mixing bowls:** No kitchen is complete without a set of good mixing bowls, and stainless-steel bowls are the most durable. The nonstick rubber base gives stability, making blending a breeze. A set of three sizes is perfect to meet all your needs, and they nest together for efficient storage.

» **A slow cooker:** Nothing spells convenience like a slow cooker. What's great is you can usually leave a slow cooker unattended all day. You put recipe ingredients in it before you leave for work and voila! You come home to a meal! A slow cooker meal is an excellent choice for a busy day, whether you work in or out of your home.

TIP

» Whenever you purchase a new slow cooker, use it a few times on both *high* and *low* settings before leaving it unattended.

» **A stainless-steel colander:** Talk about convenience, a good colander is truly an essential kitchen tool. Use it to drain water from pasta or steam veggies or to wash veggies. Because you'll be eating a lot of veggies, a colander is one kitchen tool you can't do without.

TIP

» Using stainless colanders allow them to double as a veggie steamer over a pot of boiling water. This steamer hack is as simple as it gets. Just place your food in your colander and place it on top of your pot of water. You can also store colanders in pots so they don't take up a lot of kitchen space!

» **An avocado slicer:** Avocado is one of the healthiest foods on earth, but the idea of cutting, slicing, peeling, and pitting one is a daunting task. Introducing the avocado slicer, a simple kitchen tool that makes removing the pit and slicing the fruit evenly, super easy.

» **A grater and zester:** Graters and zesters are fantastic for adding that extra flavor profile to your meals. A grater has larger holes than a zester and cuts things into ribbons or strands. Graters are wonderful for shredding cheese or garnishing with citrus peels. A zester is a must-have tool for creating a sprinkle effect, not quite like the shreds a grater does. Using a zester is much more practical than a grater, if you only need a small pinch of an ingredient such as fresh lime or lemon skin zest.

>> **A can opener:** You don't need to invest in an electric one that can take up valuable counter space. A good manual opener is absolutely essential for opening all your beans and tomato products with ease. Buy a highly rated manual can opener, one without gimmicky bonus features and made with metal not plastic.

>> **A salad spinner:** Because you'll be eating lots of darky leafy vegetables, a good salad spinner is another time saving device. You can use your colander, but a salad spinner is much more efficient. A salad spinner is the answer to your salad problems because it will help you get rid of water in a matter of seconds and save on paper towels. You can also use this tool to dry fresh herbs.

Boning Up on the Healthiest Cooking Techniques

Plant-based diets consist of eating, well, lots of plants. Plant foods contain significant amounts of natural plant chemicals that provide desirable health benefits beyond basic nutrition and reduce the risk of diseases such as cancer and cardiovascular disease. The vividly colored fruits and vegetables are known to be good sources of these free-radical-scavenging, life-extending plant chemicals known scientifically as *bioactive compounds.* How you cook plant foods has a significant effect on the retention of the antioxidant activity of these bioactive compounds.

There is a plethora of ways to cook juicy and flavorful food, but using the healthiest techniques — ones where the food still tastes delicious but where the food retains its nutrition — is just as important. More than likely you know that deep frying probably isn't the leanest cooking style, but what you may not know is how you cook your food affects the food's nutritional value. For example, boiling broccoli or spinach will result in a loss of up to 50 percent or more of their vitamin C content. With other foods, heat can amplify the release of nutrients. With carrots, and tomatoes, for example, heat breaks down cell walls, facilitating the release of antioxidants (*lycopene* in tomatoes and *carotenoids* in carrots) into the body.

As a result, you want to select the right cooking method to maximize the nutritional quality of your meal. The following sections give an overview of different cooking methods and their pros and cons.

REMEMBER

There is no perfect cooking method that retains all nutrients. In general, cooking for shorter periods at lower temperatures with minimal water will produce the best results. Don't let the nutrients in your food go down the drain!

Microwave cooking

Microwave cooking is one of the better techniques for protecting nutrients in food. That's because the short cooking times and reduced exposure to heat preserve more of the vitamins, minerals, and antioxidants in food than other cooking methods. Microwaves cook food from the inside out, the waves cause the generation of heat from the molecules moving around within the food. Microwaving broccoli, for example, results in a loss of 20 percent of the vitamin C compared to 50 percent in boiling.

Roasting and baking

These cooking techniques refer to cooking food in an oven with dry heat. Most vitamin losses are minimal with these two techniques, including vitamin C, making roasting perfect for preparing your veggies (drizzled with extra-virgin olive oil [EVOO]).

Boiling

Boiling, simmering, and poaching are similar methods of water-based cooking. These techniques differ by water temperature, boiling is hottest (212° F). Water-based cooking is fine for pasta but causes the greatest loss of vitamin C found in vegetables. (Poaching fish is fine because it doesn't cause any losses of healthy omega-3 fat or other nutrients.)

WARNING

The cooking method most destructive to heat-sensitive vitamin C and the B vitamins is boiling.

Grilling

Grilling is when the heat source comes from the bottom, compared to broiling, where the heat comes from the top. Grilling is one of the most popular cooking methods because of the great flavor it gives food. Grilling requires minimal added fats and imparts a smoky flavor while keeping food juicy and tender. Not only can grilling be a healthy and fun way to cook, if done correctly, but it also can save you tons of calories and make those high nutrient foods, oh so flavorful.

REMEMBER

The main drawback is the potential for the formation of carcinogens. However, you can do several things to help reduce the formation of carcinogenic heterocyclic amines (HA) and polycyclic aromatic hydrocarbons (PAH). These proven carcinogens are chemicals formed when food, especially fatty foods such as meats, are placed in contact with intense heat and flame for a prolonged period of time. Studies have shown that HA and PAH formation can be lessened and even prevented.

Follow these five tips for safe grilling and enjoy the flavor and health benefits of cooking in this favorite American cooking pastime:

>> **Precook meats.** The less contact with high heat and flames the food has the less chance for the formation of carcinogens. Try precooking chicken in the microwave for a minute or so to lessen cooking time on the grill.

>> **Use low-fat meats and trim excess fat.** The key word in healthful grilling is *low-fat*. That's because the fat is what causes the problems, so eating lean is your best bet. Trim all visible fat off meats and poultry or better yet, eat lean fish or shellfish.

>> **Use marinades.** Marinating low-fat foods not only adds flavor but it's also a great way to prevent the formation of HA and PAH. The best marinade choice is an EVOO, citrus, and herb concoction (think lemon juice, rosemary, basil, or thyme). EVOO provides a healthful outer shield to foods; herbs and citrus provide antioxidants that have been scientifically proven to reduce carcinogen formation.

>> **Avoid flare-ups.** Flame flare-ups (such as when the fire erupts engulfing food in flames) burn foods, increasing the formation of carcinogenic compounds.

>> **Don't char foods.** Charring foods, especially meats, isn't smart. The small areas of char are actually the most highly concentrated sources of HA and PAH, so cut off the charred sections of your BBQ and toss them.

Sautéing and stir-frying

With sautéing and stir-frying, food is cooked in a sauté pan or wok over medium to high heat in a small amount of oil. These techniques are very similar, but with stir-frying, the food is stirred often, the temperature is higher, and the cooking time is shorter. Both methods are healthy as long as you sparingly use oil, preferably EVOO. The shorter the cooking time and heat exposure, the more nutrients preserved, so stir-frying is the better of the two.

Steaming

Steaming is the best cooking method for retaining nutrients in food. Research shows that steaming vegetables such as broccoli and spinach reduce vitamin C content by only approximately 10 percent. The downside is that steamed vegetables may taste bland. However, an easy remedy is to add some seasonings and a spritz of butter spray.

Utilizing Additional Tips And Tricks to Maximize Nutrient Retention

Proponents of the raw food diet believe that eating raw foods can improve their health, wellbeing, and possibly reduce the risk of medical conditions.

WARNING

However, some foods aren't safe to eat uncooked. The cooking process breaks down toxic chemicals in some food, and others carry a risk of food poisoning. Uncooked animal products are most likely to cause food poisoning, such as raw and undercooked meat, including chicken and fish; raw or lightly cooked egg; and raw (unpasteurized) milk and products made from it. You can also get food poisoning from raw fruits and vegetables, although that's less likely with cooked fruits and vegetables because the cooking process kills bacteria. Always wash produce under running water before eating it.

Cooking food will always lead to some nutrient losses. However, you can reduce the destruction of healthful vitamins and minerals when cooking your food by using these strategies:

>> Prepare food only when it's about to be eaten; where possible eat it raw.

>> Use as little water as possible when poaching or boiling.

>> Use cooking methods that reduce cooking time duration. Refer to the section, "Boning Up on the Healthiest Cooking Techniques," earlier in this chapter.

>> Cut fruit up right before eating, such as cantaloupe, to preserve nutrients.

>> Cook vegetables in smaller amounts of water to reduce the loss of vitamin C and B vitamins; steaming is better.

>> Consume the liquid left in the pan after cooking vegetables.

>> Consider not peeling vegetables and just scrubbing them to maximize their fiber and nutrient density. Whenever possible, leave the skin on when cooking them.

>> Try to eat any cooked vegetables within a day or two, because their vitamin C content may continue to decline when the cooked food is exposed to air.

>> Cut food after — rather than before — cooking, if possible. When food is cooked whole, less of it is exposed to heat and water.

>> Cook vegetables for only a few minutes whenever possible.

>> Don't use baking soda when cooking vegetables. Although it helps maintain color, vitamin C will be lost in the alkaline environment produced by baking soda.

>> When preparing food, cut into large chunks rather than small.

» **Kicking it up a notch with flavorful soups and salads**

» **Focusing on the main course**

» **Saving room for desserts and snacks**

Chapter **21**

Starting Your Healthy Recipe Collection

Welcome to the world of nutritious cooking, the perfect complement to your intermittent fasting plan. Cooking with fresh seafood, vegetables, fruits, and grains forms the foundation of your healthy eating plan. For the best flavor and results when creating or following the recipes in this chapter, here are some helpful recommendations:

» **Fresh seafood (fish fillets, mussels, scallops, and shrimp):** If frozen fish or shrimp is used, thaw them completely before proceeding. When cooking the fish, remember most fish fillets need to cook about 10 minutes per inch of thickness to be fully cooked.

» **Salt:** Try kosher salt instead of table salt for a clean flavor and salt that readily dissolves. Per teaspoon, kosher salt contains about half the amount of sodium than table salt due to the larger size of the salt crystals. You can always use less salt than specified in the recipes, but the amount of kosher salt is a guideline for how to get the best flavor with the minimal amount of sodium. You can also use a coarse grain sea salt, if you prefer — just be sure to use just a smidgeon.

» **Broths:** Always use reduced-sodium chicken or vegetable broths.

» **Herbs:** Always use fresh chopped herbs unless otherwise specified for better flavor.

» **Citrus:** Always use freshly squeezed lemons or limes and orange juice.

» **Garlic cloves:** Use fresh medium-sized cloves of garlic, peeled, and then minced or chopped.

» **Black pepper:** Use freshly ground black pepper.

» **White wine:** Use white wine you would drink, like Chardonnay, and not a cooking wine.

» **Extra-virgin olive oil (EVOO):** Use an authentic EVOO in all recipes.

» **Canned beans:** Use low-sodium canned beans that are drained and rinsed.

» **Basic marinade formula:** Use 1-part vinegar plus 3-parts EVOO plus seasonings.

Serving Up Appetizers for Intermittent Fasting

Take the edge off your hunger by starting your eating window with these light and easy recipes for appetizers or a light meal. Treat yourself to these healthy starters that pack flavor — not calories. If you aren't in the mood to cook your appetizers, having a plate of chopped vegetables (called *crudités*) served with a fat-free yogurt or hummus dip, or sliced, bite-sized fruit will keep your mouth busy and your growling stomach somewhat satisfied while you prepare your main meal.

Avocado Shrimp Ceviche

PREP TIME: 10 MIN	COOK TIME: 0 MIN	YIELD: 8 SERVINGS

INGREDIENTS

1 pound of raw jumbo shrimp (peeled)

¼ cup fresh lime juice

½ red onion, chopped

¼ cup fresh cilantro, minced

½ teaspoon ground black pepper

¼ teaspoon salt

2 ripe avocados (about 1 cup)

DIRECTIONS

1 Cut the tails off the shrimp and discard. Chop the shrimp into ½-inch pieces and place in a large bowl.

2 Add the lime juice, red onion, cilantro, pepper, and salt, and toss to combine. Cover and refrigerate for at least 1 hour or up to 4 hours.

3 Just before serving, peel the avocado and in a separate bowl mash with a fork creating a paste. Add to the ceviche, and gently toss to combine.

PER SERVING: *Calories 140; Total fat: 7g; Saturated fat: 1.5g; Cholesterol: 115mg; Sodium: 240mg; Carbohydrates: 5g; Fiber: 4g; Sugar: 0g; Protein: 15g.*

NOTE: Fresh cilantro is the leaf from the coriander plant. Cilantro is the key ingredient to add just enough zest to your ceviche.

Garlic Bruschetta Bread

PREP TIME: 5 MIN	COOK TIME: 10 MIN	YIELD: 10 SERVINGS (SLICES)

INGREDIENTS

1 cup tomatoes, diced

2 garlic cloves, grated

2 tablespoons fresh basil, chopped

2 teaspoons extra-virgin olive oil

Pinch lemon zest

Juice from one lemon

Pinch sea salt

Pinch black pepper

1 commercial whole grain French bread loaf, 12 oz

DIRECTIONS

1 In a small bowl, combine the tomatoes, garlic, basil, 1 teaspoon of olive oil, lemon zest, lemon juice, salt, and pepper, and set aside for at least 15 minutes to let the flavors marry for a bit.

2 Preheat oven to 450° F.

3 Slice the bread on a diagonal into ten slices. Place the bread slices on a lightly oiled baking sheet. Drizzle slices with the remaining olive oil.

4 Bake the bread until golden brown for 8 to 10 minutes.

5 Mound the bread slices with the bruschetta mixture and serve.

PER SERVING: *Calories 110; Total fat: 3g; Saturated fat: 0 g; Cholesterol: 0 mg; Sodium: 190mg; Carbohydrates: 18g; Fiber: 1 g; Sugar: 0g; Protein: 3g.*

TIP: Keep an eye on the bread in the oven. Slices should be golden.

Eggplant Dip

INGREDIENTS

1 large eggplant (about 1½ pounds)

2 garlic cloves, peeled and chopped

¼ cup chopped flat-leaf parsley

Juice of 1 lemon

1 tablespoon tahini

¼ teaspoon kosher salt

¼ teaspoon cayenne pepper

2 tablespoons extra-virgin olive oil

DIRECTIONS

1 Preheat oven to 450° F.

2 Using a fork, prick the eggplant in about eight places. Place on a foil-lined baking sheet. Bake for 35 to 40 minutes or until soft. Remove from the oven and let cool.

3 Cut the eggplant in half, drain any liquid, and scoop out the pulp into a blender or food processor. Add the garlic, parsley, lemon juice, tahini, salt, cayenne pepper, and olive oil.

4 Blend until smooth. Refrigerate for 30 minutes to blend flavors.

PER SERVING: *Calories 77; Total fat: 6g; Saturated fat: 1g; Cholesterol: 0mg; Sodium: 50mg; Carbohydrates: 6g; Fiber: 3g; Sugar: 2g; Protein: 1g.*

TIP: For a smoky flavor, cook your eggplant on the grill. Be sure to eliminate as much moisture as possible and add your oil slowly into blender.

Roasted Eggplant Tomato Stack

PREP TIME: 10 MIN	COOK TIME: 60 MIN	YIELD: 6 SERVINGS

INGREDIENTS

1 medium eggplant, sliced into ¾- to 1-inch slices

⅛ cup extra-virgin olive oil

1 large steak tomato, 6 slices

½ cup of goat cheese, crumbled

Balsamic Caramelized Onions

¼ cup extra virgin olive oil

2 yellow onions, thinly sliced

¼ cup brown sugar

⅔ cup aged balsamic vinegar

¼ cup aged balsamic vinegar

DIRECTIONS

1 Preheat oven to 350° F.

2 On a baking sheet, place the sliced eggplant. Pour ⅛ cup of olive oil in a small bowl and brush both sides of the eggplant slices with oil. Roast the eggplant slices for 45 minutes (flip slices over every 15 minutes).

3 While the eggplant is roasting, make the onions. In a medium skillet over medium heat, heat the olive oil. Add the onions, stirring often, until they start to soften (about 10 minutes). Add the brown sugar and ⅔ cup balsamic vinegar to the frying pan and stir. Reduce heat to medium low and continue to cook, stirring often, until deep golden and a jam–like consistency, 45 to 60 minutes.

4 Remove the onions from pan and pour ¼ cup balsamic vinegar. As the liquid bubbles, scrape the browned and caramelized bits and mix into glaze. Reserve glaze to pour over stacks.

5 To create the stack, you'll need 12 slices of eggplant and 6 slices of tomato. Layer one eggplant slice, 1 tomato slice, ⅛ cup of onions, 1 eggplant slice, ⅛ cup of onions, a sprinkle of goat cheese, and 2 tablespoons of balsamic glaze (bottom to top).

PER SERVING: *Calories 237; Total fat: 12g; Saturated fat: 2g; Cholesterol: 7mg; Sodium: 66mg; Carbohydrates: 28g; Fiber: 6g; Sugar: 2g; Protein: 5g.*

TIP: You can't rush true caramelized onions. Making them at home is simple but requires patience. The sugars trapped inside the onion layers caramelize steadily with time and a medium-low heat.

Savoring Salads, Soups, and Sandwiches

Filling up on fiber- and water-rich soups and salads before your main meal can help you lose weight without severely restricting food and caloric intake. The high water and fiber content in soups and veggie-rich salads fills you up to prevent hunger cravings that lead to overeating. Fill your soups and salads with a variety of nutrient-rich, low-calorie foods including vegetables and legumes.

In addition, sandwiches are a perfect go-to food if you want a quick and healthy nutrient-packed light meal during your eating window. If you're out and about during your eating window, you may consider throwing a shelf-stable whole-grain peanut butter and banana sandwich into your purse or gym bag.

TIP

Keep frozen whole-grain pita breads, 100 percent whole-grain burger buns, and veggie burgers in your freezer. For a quick and nutritious meal in minutes, make a veggie burger topped with spinach, tomato, onions, avocado, and a pesto spread.

Watermelon Feta Salad

PREP TIME: 10 MIN	COOK TIME: 0 MIN	YIELD: 2 SERVINGS

INGREDIENTS

4 cups red leaf lettuce, washed, dried, and torn

¼ cup crumbled feta

2 cups watermelon, cubed

¼ red onion, sliced

½ cup yellow grape tomatoes, sliced in half

½ cup of cucumber, chopped

Balsamic Dressing

¾ cup extra-virgin olive oil

¼ cup aged balsamic vinegar

1 tablespoon Dijon mustard

1 shallot, peeled and minced

1 bunch flat-leaf Italian parsley, stalks removed

3 stalks fresh chives, cut into small pieces

DIRECTIONS

1 Rinse, dry, and cut up the vegetables as directed. Mix all the ingredients in a large bowl.

2 To make the dressing, place all the ingredients in a blender. Blend until well combined, scraping down the sides of the container at least once. Use 2 tablespoons to dress your salad and serve immediately. Refrigerate leftover dressing for later use.

PER SERVING: *Calories 128; Total fat: 4g; Saturated fat: 2g; Cholesterol: 13mg; Sodium: 222mg; Carbohydrates: 16g; Fiber: 2g; Sugar: 0g; Protein: 6g.*

SALAD DRESSING: *Calories 123; Total fat: 14g; Saturated fat: 2g; Cholesterol: 0mg; Sodium: 18mg; Carbohydrates: 1g; Fiber: 0g; Sugar: 0g; Protein: 0g.*

TIP: For the balsamic vinaigrette, use a well-aged balsamic vinegar. It's delicious served on a salad, a fillet of fish, or as a marinade for roasting vegetables. Dressing can be stored in the refrigerator up to three days. If you prefer a more acidic vinaigrette, increase the vinegar to ½ cup.

NOTE: The yield for the dressing in this recipe is 12 servings.

Citrus Asian Tempeh Salad

PREP TIME: 20 MIN | **COOK TIME: 10 MIN** | **YIELD: 2 SERVINGS**

INGREDIENTS

4 tablespoons orange juice

1 tablespoon teriyaki stir fry sauce

6 ounces tempeh, soy, uncooked (¾ of a typical 8-ounce package)

2 tablespoons extra-virgin olive oil

5 cups assorted mixed salad greens (spinach, arugula, endive, radicchio)

½ cup edamame (shelled)

1 navel orange, slivered

2 tablespoons slivered almonds

Citrus Vinaigrette

¾ cup apple cider vinegar

3 tablespoons fresh lemon juice

3 tablespoons fresh orange juice

1 tablespoon honey

1 garlic clove, minced

Dash sea salt

Dash fresh ground black pepper

¼ cup extra-virgin olive oil

DIRECTIONS

1 In a small bowl, mix the orange juice with the teriyaki stir fry sauce.

2 Cut the uncooked tempeh into eight to ten slices or cubes and place in a second small bowl. Add the marinade to the tempeh and mix well. Let tempeh sit in marinade for 15 minutes.

3 Add the oil to skillet. Cook the tempeh on medium for about 5 minutes on both sides or until the tempeh is golden brown and crispy.

4 In a large salad bowl, add the greens, edamame, and orange.

5 In a small bowl, whisk all the ingredients together, slowing adding in the olive oil. Add the cooked tempeh and 4 tablespoons of the citrus vinaigrette in the salad bowl and mix well. Use the vinaigrette to dress your salad and refrigerate the extra for later use.

PER SERVING: *Calories 580; Total fat: 36g; Saturated fat: 6g; Cholesterol: 0 mg; Sodium: 280mg; Carbohydrates: 45g; Fiber: 6g; Sugar: 23g; Protein: 26g.*

TIP: Slicing tempeh to about a ¼-inch thickness is ideal for acquiring just the right amount of crispiness on the edges while retaining a nice, chewy interior.

TIP: Dressing can be stored in the refrigerator up to three days.

Tuna Salad with Tofu

PREP TIME: 20 MIN	COOK TIME: 0 MIN	YIELD: 2 SERVINGS

INGREDIENTS

4 cups red leaf lettuce, washed, dried, and torn

One 14-ounce package extra firm tofu

1 large ripe tomato, diced

½ large Vidalia sweet onion, sliced

½ cup sliced button mushrooms

One 12-ounce can of water packed tuna fish

¼ cup scallions, sliced (green part only)

Dressing

1 clove garlic, minced

1 tablespoon balsamic vinegar (well-aged)

1½ teaspoons Dijon mustard

⅛ teaspoon salt

⅛ teaspoon freshly ground black pepper

⅓ cup extra virgin olive oil

DIRECTIONS

1 Arrange the lettuce on a large salad plate. Cut the tofu into one-inch cubes and add to the salad. Add the tomato, onion, and mushroom together and sprinkle over the tofu. Sprinkle the drained tuna flakes over the tomato mixture and then add the green onions.

2 In a small bowl, whisk together all the dressing ingredients except the oil and blend until smooth. Slowly add in the oil and mix until the dressing is a thick consistency. Chill until serving salad.

3 Pour the chilled dressing over the salad before serving.

PER SERVING: *Calories 461; Total fat: 17g; Saturated fat: 1g; Cholesterol: 51 mg; Sodium: 779mg; Carbohydrates: 15g; Fiber: 2g; Sugar: 7g; Protein: 60g.*

TIP: When working with extra-firm tofu, press the tofu to get as much water out as possible. If you don't have a press, use paper towels around the block, place on a plate, add a second plate, and press. Change the paper towels and repeat. The longer it sits, pressed, the better.

Couscous Red Bean Salad

PREP TIME: 20 MIN	COOK TIME: 10 MIN	YIELD: 4 SERVINGS

INGREDIENTS

1⅓ cups reduced-sodium chicken or vegetable broth

½ teaspoon salt

1 cup uncooked couscous, preferably whole grain

1 tablespoon extra-virgin olive oil

2 tablespoons freshly squeezed lemon juice

1 teaspoon red wine vinegar

1 teaspoon ground cumin

¼ teaspoon cayenne powder

Two 15-ounce cans of low-sodium dark red kidney beans, rinsed and drained

½ cup scallions, whites and greens, sliced (4 scallions)

¾ cup red bell pepper, seeded and chopped

¾ cup yellow bell pepper, seeded and chopped

2 tablespoons fresh cilantro, chopped

Salt and pepper to taste

DIRECTIONS

1 In a medium saucepan, bring the broth to a boil.

2 Remove the pan from the heat and pour in the salt and couscous. Stir to evenly moisten the couscous.

3 Cover the pan and let it sit for 10 minutes or until all the broth is absorbed and the couscous is tender. Fluff the couscous with a fork and set aside.

4 In a small bowl, whisk together the olive oil, lemon juice, red wine vinegar, ground cumin, and cayenne powder. Set aside.

5 Place the couscous in a large salad-serving bowl. Add the kidney beans, scallions, bell peppers, and cilantro. Toss with the dressing. Season with salt and pepper. Let the salad sit for 20 to 30 minutes for all the flavors to blend well together. Serve at room temperature.

PER SERVING: *Calories 490; Total fat: 6g; Saturated fat: 1 g; Cholesterol: 0 mg; Sodium: 880 mg; Carbohydrates: 87g; Fiber: 1g; Sugar: 11g; Protein: 24g.*

TIP: This is a great make-ahead salad. Cook up to 24 hours before, add the dressing, and let marinate. Just be sure to hold off adding the cilantro until right before serving.

Bulgur Wheat Citrus Salad

PREP TIME: 10 MIN	COOK TIME: 10 MIN	YIELD: 4 SERVINGS

INGREDIENTS

1 cup bulgur wheat

¾ cup frozen, shelled edamame (soya) beans

2 Romano peppers, sliced into rounds, seeded

¾ cup radish, finely sliced

⅓ cup almonds, sliced

¼ cup mint, finely chopped

¼ cup parsley, finely chopped

2 navel oranges

3 tablespoon extra-virgin olive oil

¼ teaspoon salt

¼ teaspoon freshly ground black pepper

DIRECTIONS

1 Cook the bulgur wheat following the instructions on the package. After it's finished, drain and transfer to a large mixing bowl.

2 Place the edamame beans in a small bowl and pour in a cup of boiling water to cook. Let beans sit in water for 1 minute, then drain.

3 Transfer the edamame to the serving bowl with the bulgur wheat. Add in the sliced peppers, radish, almonds, mint, and parsley.

4 Peel one orange and cut into ½-inch pieces. Juice the second orange. Transfer the orange juice into a jam jar along with the olive oil. Add a pinch of salt and pepper, cover the jar, and shake to emulsify dressing. Pour the dressing over the salad mixture and serve.

PER SERVING: *Calories 380; Total fat: 18g; Saturated fat: 2g; Cholesterol: 0mg; Sodium: 230mg; Carbohydrates: 47g; Fiber: 12g; Sugar: 8g; Protein: 12g.*

TIP: For less spice, swap Romano peppers for a red bell pepper.

Split Pea Soup

PREP TIME: 10 MIN	COOK TIME: 45 MIN	YIELD: 4 SERVINGS

INGREDIENTS

1 cup dried green split peas

6 cups reduced-sodium chicken broth

1 carrot, sliced

1 Vidalia onion, quartered

Pinch dried leaf marjoram

Pinch dried leaf thyme

Dash red cayenne pepper

1 teaspoon imitation bacon bits

Drizzle extra-virgin olive oil

DIRECTIONS

1 Rinse the split peas.

2 In a large saucepan, place all the ingredients except the bacon bits and oil into saucepan and bring to a boil. Cover, reduce heat, and simmer 45 minutes until tender. Remove from heat.

3 After they're cooled, process in a blender or a food processor fitted with a metal blade. Process to a smooth consistency.

4 Return to a saucepan to warm before serving; add the bacon bits and a drizzle of extra-virgin olive oil immediately before serving.

PER SERVING: *Calories 230; Total fat: 2.5g; Saturated fat: 0 g; Cholesterol: 0 mg; Sodium: 660 mg; Carbohydrates: 38g; Fiber: 13g; Sugar: 8g; Protein: 14g.*

TIP: The great thing about cooking with split peas, as opposed to many other types of dried legumes, is that they require zero soaking. The 45-minute simmer will cook them well, and they'll start to break down and thicken the soup.

Lentil Soup

PREP TIME: 10 MIN	COOK TIME: 30 MIN	YIELD: 9 SERVINGS

INGREDIENTS

1½ tablespoons extra-virgin olive oil

1½ large Vidalia onions, diced (about 2 cups)

5 carrots, peeled and diced (about 2 cups)

5 garlic cloves, peeled and chopped

2 cups brown lentils, rinsed and picked over

One 15-ounce can diced tomatoes

¼ cup tomato paste

1 tablespoon curry powder

1 tablespoon sweet paprika

6 cups reduced-sodium chicken broth

1 cup fresh parsley, chopped

1 cup fresh cilantro, chopped

½ teaspoon hot sauce

Drizzle extra virgin olive oil (if desired)

Sprinkle of Parmesan cheese (if desired)

DIRECTIONS

1 In a large soup pot, heat the olive oil over medium heat.

2 Add the onions, carrots, and garlic and cook until softened and golden, about 10 minutes. Stir in the lentils, tomatoes, tomato paste, curry powder, paprika, and chicken broth. Cook for 30 minutes, until lentils are soft, stirring frequently. Add the parsley, cilantro, and hot sauce.

3 Serve hot and top with a drizzle of extra-virgin olive oil and shredded Parmesan cheese if desired.

PER SERVING: *Calories 230; Total fat: 3.5 g; Saturated fat: 0 g; Cholesterol: 0 mg; Sodium: 350 mg; Carbohydrates: 39 g; Fiber: 7g; Sugar: 8 g; Protein: 13g.*

TIP: To make this a vegan soup, use vegetable broth in lieu of chicken broth.

Lentil Falafel Pita Sandwich

PREP TIME: 45 MIN	COOK TIME: 35 MIN	YIELD: 4 SERVINGS

INGREDIENTS

4 cups water

1 cup lentils, rinsed and picked over

1 onion, finely chopped

1 carrot, diced

¾ teaspoon salt

1 tablespoon curry powder

1 teaspoon ground cumin

⅓ cup whole wheat seasoned breadcrumbs

1 large egg white

4 tablespoons extra-virgin olive oil (or more as needed)

2 whole wheat pita

½ cucumber, sliced

1 large beef tomato, sliced

½ red onion, sliced

1 cup red leaf lettuce, torn

Tahini

4 tablespoons tahini paste

3 fresh garlic cloves

Drizzle extra virgin olive oil

Juice from 1 lemon, divided

Yogurt Sauce

6-ounce container nonfat Greek yogurt

1 garlic clove, chopped

1 tablespoon fresh dill, stems removed, chopped

DIRECTIONS

1 In a medium saucepan combine the water, lentils, onion, carrot, and ½ teaspoon salt and bring to a boil over medium-high heat. Stir and simmer covered for 30 minutes. Drain and cool.

2 By hand, combine the lentil mixture, the remaining salt, spices, breadcrumbs, and egg white. Shape the falafel mixture into small, round, flattened patties (approximately 1-inch rounds). Heat 2 tablespoons oil in a large skillet (swirl to coat pan), until the oil is hot enough that a droplet of water sizzles. Fry in batches, adding more oil as necessary, until golden brown on all sides (approximately 3 to 5 minutes). Remove and place on paper towels to soak up excess oil.

3 For tahini, in a food processor, add the tahini paste, garlic cloves and a drizzle of olive oil and lemon juice and blend. For yogurt sauce, blend by hand the chopped garlic clove with nonfat Greek yogurt, a drizzle olive oil, and a squeeze of fresh lemon juice. Top with chopped fresh dill.

4 To make your sandwich, cut one whole wheat pita bread in half to make two half-pockets. Pour two tablespoons of tahini sauce inside each pita half. Fill each pocket with two falafel patties, two cucumber slices, 2 tomato slices, 1 slice red onion, and as much lettuce as desired. Top with the yogurt sauce and serve.

PER SERVING: *Calories 428; Total fat: 21g; Saturated fat: 2g; Cholesterol: 1mg; Sodium: 607mg; Carbohydrates: 50g; Fiber: 8g; Sugar: 7g; Protein: 14g.*

TIP: Use commercial tahini sauce and a dollop of plain nonfat Greek yogurt if you don't want to make the sauce from scratch.

Portobello Mushroom Burgers

PREP TIME: 20 MIN	COOK TIME: 10 MIN	YIELD: 4 SERVINGS

INGREDIENTS

4 Portobello mushrooms, rinsed, stem and gills removed

2 red peppers, washed, cored, seeded, and halved

4 whole wheat burger buns

2 cups fresh arugula

4 tablespoons pesto

Marinade

¼ cup extra-virgin olive oil

2 tablespoons balsamic vinegar

½ teaspoon salt

¼ teaspoon freshly ground black pepper

¼ cup fresh parsley leaves, chopped

2 garlic cloves, minced

DIRECTIONS

1 Spray your grill with nonstick spray, and preheat it to medium-hot heat (about 400° F).

2 In a medium bowl, whisk together the marinade ingredients: oil, vinegar, salt, pepper, parsley, and garlic.

3 Brush the marinade on both sides of the mushroom caps and peppers and let them sit for 10 minutes.

4 Place the peppers, skin side up, on the hot grill rack. Cover the grill and cook the peppers 4 to 5 minutes or until beginning to soften. Turn the peppers over; cover and cook 3 to 4 minutes longer or until slightly charred. As peppers are done, return them to the marinade bowl. Add parsley and toss to coat.

5 Remove the mushrooms from the bowl, shaking off any excess marinade and reserving the marinade for basting. Cook on each side for 5 to 7 minutes, or until caramelized and deep golden brown. Brush the remaining marinade over the mushrooms several times as they cook.

6 Place the grilled mushroom cap, bell pepper, and ½ cup arugula on one half of burger bun. Spread heart-healthy pesto on the other half of the bun as a condiment.

PER SERVING: *Calories 330; Total fat: 17g; Saturated fat: 2.5g; Cholesterol: 0mg; Sodium: 650mg; Carbohydrates: 41g; Fiber: 3g; Sugar: 7g; Protein: 11g.*

TIP: Pesto is a healthier alternative than sugar-laden ketchup for topping your burgers. You could also use Dijon mustard as a spread in lieu of the pesto. Suggested serving side: Sweet Potato Steak Fries.

Planning Plant-Based Entrees for Intermittent Fasting

Eating more plants and less animals is the key to a long and healthy life. I encourage you to explore the wide world of delectable plant foods when intermittent fasting. Plant-based eating patterns focus on, well, eating lots of plants, including dark green leafy vegetables, fruit, nuts, seeds, healthy oils, whole grains, and legumes (beans, peas, and lentils).

What plant-based eating doesn't necessarily mean is that you have to become a strict vegetarian or vegan and never eat meat or dairy. Rather, you are proportionately choosing more of your foods from plant sources. Here are some definitions of a few of the plant-based eating styles you can make

>> **Vegan diet:** A vegan diet excludes all animal foods, including animal flesh, dairy products (cheese, milk, yogurt, butter), eggs, and honey.

>> **Lacto-ovo vegetarian diet:** This diet excludes all animal flesh, but it allows for dairy products and eggs.

>> **Pescatarian vegetarian diet:** This diet excludes all animal flesh, but it allows fish.

Most Americans prefer to follow a flexitarian style of eating. *Flexitarian* is a marriage of two words: flexible and vegetarian. A recent gallop poll found that U.S. consumers want to incorporate more plant-based options in their diets but are unwilling to give up animal proteins altogether. These results are in keeping with the current flurry of attention generated by the flexitarian diet.

The following recipes give you several choices and illustrate how eating a wholesome, plant-powered flexitarian diet can be easy, delicious, and extremely cost effective.

Mushroom Barley Risotto with Chicken

PREP TIME: 10 MIN	COOK TIME: 50 MIN	YIELD: 4 SERVINGS

INGREDIENTS

1 tablespoon extra-virgin olive oil

1¼ cup hulled barley

1 cup white wine

1 cup reduced-sodium chicken broth

2 tablespoons extra-virgin olive oil

One 16-ounce package of sliced white mushrooms

Three 5-ounce skinless, boneless, chicken breasts, cut into large chunks

1 tablespoon fresh thyme leaves, chopped

2 large shallots, finely sliced

2 garlic cloves, chopped

Dash coarsely ground kosher salt

Dash freshly ground black pepper

½ teaspoon kosher salt

½ teaspoon freshly ground black pepper

3 tablespoons shredded Parmesan cheese

¼ cup chopped chives

DIRECTIONS

1 Heat the olive oil in a large skillet.

2 Add the barley and cook for 1 minute. Pour in the wine and continually stir until the liquid absorbs. Stir in ¾ cup of chicken broth.

3 Allow the risotto to cook for 40 minutes on a low simmer and stir occasionally. Cook the barley until tender. Add the remaining chicken stock if the risotto looks dry.

4 After the risotto is almost done, cook the mushrooms and chicken breasts. Heat a large, heavy frying pan over medium-high heat and add 1 tablespoon of the olive oil. When the oil is hot, add the mushrooms and cook, stirring or tossing in the pan, for a few minutes, until they begin to soften and sweat. Add the remaining oil, turn the heat to medium, and add the thyme, shallots, garlic, salt, and pepper. Sprinkle chicken evenly on both sides with salt and pepper. Add chicken to the pan; cook 4 minutes on each side or until golden brown and done.

5 Remove the risotto pan from the heat and stir in the chicken chunks, mushrooms, and Parmesan cheese. Serve immediately, adding chopped chives and Parmesan on top for garnish.

PER SERVING: *Calories 600; Total fat: 25g; Saturated fat: 7g; Cholesterol: 30mg; Sodium: 740mg; Carbohydrates: 45g; Fiber: 1g; Sugar: 6g; Protein: 17g.*

TIP: While cooking, the risotto should continually be stirred at least every 3 to 5 minutes to ensure that the barley soaks up the liquid. Chewy and rich in fiber, hulled barley is the healthiest kind of barley compared to pearl; however, it takes longer to cook.

Zucchini Pizza

PREP TIME: 10 MIN	COOK TIME: 40 MIN	YIELD: 4 SERVINGS

INGREDIENTS

1 16-ounce whole wheat pizza dough

2 cups sliced zucchini (about 1 large)

1 Vidalia onion, sliced crosswise

3 tablespoons extra-virgin olive oil

Pinch salt

Pinch freshly ground black pepper

2 cups part-skim ricotta cheese

3 tablespoons chopped fresh basil

2 tablespoons milk, 1 percent

1–2 teaspoons fresh lemon juice

4 garlic cloves, minced

4 ounces goat cheese

Crushed red pepper flakes and fresh watercress

DIRECTIONS

1 Preheat oven to 425° F. Take the dough out of the fridge and let it come to room temperature. Toss the zucchini and onion with 2 tablespoons of oil on a rimmed parchment-lined baking sheet; season with the salt and pepper. Lay zucchini slices and onion in an even layer, spread out across the pan. Roast on top rack, tossing with a spatula once halfway through, until vegetables are browned all over and tender, about 20 minutes. Let cool.

2 Place the dough in the center of another large baking sheet and drizzle with 1 tablespoon oil and then turn to coat. Pick up the dough and stretch it out with your hands, rotating it and working from the center toward the outer edges, before placing it on the baking sheet. Keep stretching it until you've formed a rough rectangle. Make sure the dough is as even as possible. Poke the dough with a fork and season with salt. Bake the dough on the bottom rack for about 15 minutes, until slightly crispy.

3 Whisk the ricotta, basil, milk, lemon juice, and garlic together in a medium bowl. You can use a mixer if needed. Add the salt and pepper to taste. Spread half of the ricotta mixture onto the dough, and then top with the zucchini. Finish by crumbling the goat cheese on top.

4 Bake for 10 to 15 minutes or until the crust and toppings are browned to your liking. Remove from the oven and sprinkle with crushed red pepper, watercress, and freshly ground pepper if you prefer. Slice and serve warm.

PER SERVING: *Calories 570; Total fat: 22g; Saturated fat: 8g; Cholesterol: 40 mg; Sodium: 840mg; Carbohydrates: 64g; Fiber: 1g; Sugar: 13g; Protein: 26g.*

TIP: Prefer mozzarella cheese on your flatbread? Switch out the ricotta mixture with shredded part-skim mozzarella for a cheesier pizza.

NOTE: When stretching the dough, it's okay if it doesn't fill the entire baking sheet.

Tomato Arugula Flatbread

PREP TIME: 30 MIN	COOK TIME: 15 MIN	YIELD: 6 SERVINGS

INGREDIENTS

⅔ cup warm water

1 teaspoon salt

¼ cup extra-virgin olive oil

2 cups white whole wheat flour

8 ounces grape tomatoes

6 ounces fresh mozzarella cheese

½ cup pesto

4 ounces walnuts, chopped

Salad

2 tablespoons well-aged balsamic vinegar

½ teaspoon honey

½ teaspoon Dijon mustard

½ shallot, minced

1 garlic clove, minced

Dash salt

Dash black pepper

¼ cup extra-virgin olive oil

One 5-ounce container organic baby arugula

DIRECTIONS

1 Combine the warm water and salt until the salt dissolves. Stir in the olive oil. Add in the whole wheat flour and work it with your hands until the moisture is distributed and you make a soft, elastic, slightly sticky dough. Knead the dough on a lightly floured work surface until it's smooth, about 1 minute. Divide the dough into six pieces and shape them each into a ball. Cover the dough balls and allow them to rest for about 15 minutes. Spray a skillet with nonstick olive oil spray. Spread out or flatten each dough ball into a flat, rectangle–like shape. Heat each flatbread in a pan over medium heat for 2 to 3 minutes per side. Let cool.

2 Preheat oven to 450° F. Place the flatbreads on a baking sheet lined with parchment paper. Halve the tomatoes and thinly slice the mozzarella. Spread each flatbread with a thin layer of pesto. Top with slices of mozzarella and tomatoes and bake on the top rack for 5 minutes until the cheese is melted and slightly golden.

3 To make the salad, combine the balsamic vinegar, honey, Dijon mustard, shallot, garlic, salt, and black pepper together in a mixing bowl. Slowly whisk in the olive oil. Dress the arugula salad. Top the flatbread with the arugula salad and walnuts and serve.

PER SERVING: *Calories 610; Total fat: 46g; Saturated fat: 9g; Cholesterol: 20 mg; Sodium: 800mg; Carbohydrates: 40g; Fiber: 6g; Sugar: 5g; Protein: 17g.*

TIP: Give flatbreads additional flavor by whisking in ½ to 1 teaspoon fresh or dried herbs: rosemary, oregano, basil, and thyme are all delicious options. If you don't want to make flatbread from scratch, substitute a commercial whole wheat pizza dough.

Eggplant Pasta

PREP TIME: 10 MIN	COOK TIME: 70 MIN	YIELD: 8 SERVINGS

INGREDIENTS

2 pints grape tomatoes

One 1½ pound eggplant, cut into 1-inch cubes

1 cup pitted Kalamata olives

6 garlic cloves, peeled and roughly chopped

¼ cup extra-virgin olive oil

2 tablespoons fresh thyme leaves or 2 teaspoons dried

1 teaspoon kosher salt

1 teaspoon crushed red pepper flakes

½ cup thinly sliced fresh basil

1 cup fire-roasted red pepper strips

4 cups (about 8 ounces) whole-grain rotini or penne pasta

DIRECTIONS

1 Preheat oven to 375° F. Spray a rimmed baking sheet with nonstick cooking spray.

2 Place the tomatoes, eggplant, olives, and garlic on the prepared baking sheet. Drizzle with ¼ cup olive oil and season with thyme, salt, and red pepper flakes. Shake the baking sheet back and forth a few times to coat the vegetables with the oil and seasonings. Bake for 1 hour and 10 minutes until the tomatoes are softened and the eggplant is lightly browned. When the vegetables are done, remove them from the oven and spoon into them a shallow bowl or platter. Stir in the basil and red pepper strips.

3 Near the end of the cooking time for the vegetables, bring a large pot of water to a boil. Add the pasta and cook until al dente, about 10 minutes.

4 Serve the veggies over the pasta.

PER SERVING: *Calories 249; Total fat: 13 g; Saturated fat: 2 g; Cholesterol: 0 mg; Sodium: 364 mg; Carbohydrates: 32g; Fiber: 5g; Sugar: 5g; Protein: 6g.*

TIP: Roasting the tomatoes and eggplant adds a sweet, rich flavor to the vegetables — delicious served with whole-grain pasta.

NOTE: If you want, add a touch of freshly grated Parmesan cheese.

Zucchini Boats

PREP TIME: 15 MIN	COOK TIME: 40 MIN	YIELD: 4 SERVINGS

INGREDIENTS

Bruschetta

2 large tomatoes, diced

¼ cup thinly sliced basil

1 tablespoon balsamic vinegar

½ teaspoon kosher salt

Pinch crushed red pepper flakes

2 tablespoons extra-virgin olive oil

1 cloves garlic, thinly sliced

Couscous

1½ cups vegetable broth

1 tablespoon extra-virgin olive oil

1 cup couscous

2 cloves garlic, minced

1 Roma tomato, chopped

1 tablespoon Italian seasoning

Zucchini Boats

2 zucchinis

2 tablespoons extra-virgin olive oil

Pinch salt

Pinch pepper

¼ cup Parmesan cheese

½ cup mozzarella cheese

DIRECTIONS

1 In a large bowl, toss together the tomatoes, basil, balsamic vinegar, salt, and red pepper flakes. Add the garlic and oil and toss to combine. Let marinate for 30 minutes. In a medium pot, bring the vegetable broth to a boil.

2 Add oil to a skillet and heat to medium-high. Add the couscous, garlic, tomato, and ½ tablespoon of Italian seasoning. Cook and stir until fragrant, for about 1 to 2 minutes. As soon as the broth is boiling, add the couscous mixture, cover, and let sit for 5 to 10 minutes.

3 Adjust the oven by sliding one of the racks to the uppermost spot and preheat to 450° F. Wash and dry the zucchini, and then cut in half lengthwise. Scoop out the pulp and seeds with a spoon, leaving a ¼-inch-thick shell and discard the pulp. Rub each zucchini half with olive oil, and then season with salt, pepper, and remaining ½ tablespoon of Italian seasoning. Place the 4 boats on a rimmed baking pan lined with parchment.

4 Stuff the zucchini boats with couscous filling and bake for 20 minutes. Remove from the oven and top with Parmesan and mozzarella cheeses. Return the tray to the top rack of the oven and bake until the cheese melts, for approximately 3 minutes.

5 Use any remaining couscous mixture as a base for your serving plates. Top off each zucchini boat with bruschetta.

PER SERVING: *Calories 470; Total fat: 25g; Saturated fat: 7g; Cholesterol: 30mg; Sodium: 740mg; Carbohydrates: 45g; Fiber: 1g; Sugar: 6g; Protein: 17g.*

TIP: Don't scoop too much. Make sure you leave a sturdy border of zucchini flesh to support the filling.

TIP: Fluffing the couscous as it is cooks is an important step to prevent any sticking to the bottom of the pot.

Fishing for Seafood Entrees

Eating fish for a long life is called the *Eskimo factor*. As early as 1944, scientists began to document that Greenland Eskimos had virtually no heart disease (the leading cause of death in the United States). This phenomenon occurred despite the fact that the Eskimos ate a diet low in fruits, vegetables, and complex carbohydrates. But what they did subsist on was a diet loaded with oily seafood such as whale and seal meat, providing them with a huge daily dose of fish oil (about 15 grams), rich in the superbly heart-healthy, anti-inflammatory marine omega-3 fats.

REMEMBER

The best sources of omega-3 fats are the species of fish with darker meat, like salmon, mackerel, lake trout, herring, sardines, and albacore tuna. Salmon is the most affordable and richest source of omega-3 fatty acids for people living in the United States. Eat wild salmon (fresh or frozen) if you can get it; if not, farmed is perfectly fine. A reliable way to ensure that you're getting wild salmon is to buy canned Alaskan salmon. Salmon is also a low mercury fish. Mercury contamination is only a problem when high levels accumulate in the flesh of fish such as in older, larger types of predator fish such as tuna (albacore, bluefin, bigeye, and yellowfin), swordfish, marlin, and shark.

Here are some seafood recipes you can incorporate into your intermittent fasting regimen.

Teriyaki Grilled Salmon

PREP TIME: 20 MIN	COOK TIME: 10 MIN	YIELD: 8 SERVINGS

INGREDIENTS

½ cup brown sugar

4 garlic cloves, minced

1 teaspoon fresh ginger, minced

½ teaspoon red pepper flakes

1 cup less sodium soy sauce

2 tablespoons white wine

2 tablespoons extra-virgin olive oil

¼ cup scallions, chopped

2-lb wild salmon fillets (about eight 4-ounce fillets)

1 tablespoon corn starch

1 tablespoon water

DIRECTIONS

1 In a medium bowl, combine the brown sugar, garlic, ginger, red pepper flakes, soy sauce, and white wine. Reserve ½ cup and set aside into a small saucepan.

2 Add the oil and scallions to the larger marinade. Pour the marinade into a gallon sealable bag, add the salmon fillets, shake, and refrigerate for about an hour.

3 In a small bowl, create your thickening slurry by adding cornstarch and water and stir until a smooth paste forms.

4 Whisk the slurry into the reserved sauce. Cook your glaze over low heat until thickened, which should require about 5 to 10 minutes on the stovetop.

5 Grease the grill with a nonstick spray. Bring the heat of your grill to about 500° F (medium high is the best temp for grilled salmon). Place the marinated salmon fillets on top and grill until fully cooked. Salmon grill time varies depending on the thickness of the salmon fillets.

6 After the grilled salmon is cooked through completely, remove from the grill and brush the glaze on top.

PER SERVING: *Calories 310; Total fat: 15g; Saturated fat: 4 g; Cholesterol: 55 mg; Sodium: 1230 mg; Carbohydrates: 16g; Fiber: 0g; Sugar: 12g; Protein: 25g.*

TIP: You can make the teriyaki sauce a day or two ahead or time and keep it in the refrigerator until you're ready to grill.

TIP: Serve with the Couscous Red Bean Salad as a side dish.

TIP: Generally, for every 1 inch of fish, grill for about 8 minutes total (flip after 4 minutes cooking time).

NOTE: You may want to pat the salmon dry after removing it from the marinade so it allows the fish to crisp up on the skin.

Grilled Swordfish

PREP TIME: 10 MIN | COOK TIME: 10 MIN | YIELD: 2 SERVINGS

INGREDIENTS

Two 6-ounce center cut swordfish fillets

Juice of 1 lemon

3 tablespoons extra-virgin olive oil

1 garlic clove, peeled and chopped

1 tablespoon fresh chopped oregano or mint

¼ teaspoon kosher salt

½ teaspoon freshly ground black pepper

DIRECTIONS

1 Place swordfish fillets in a shallow dish.

2 Mix the lemon juice, olive oil, garlic, oregano, salt, and black pepper. Pour over the fish and refrigerate for 15 to 20 minutes.

3 Preheat a pre-sprayed grill to high heat. Grill the swordfish for about 2 minutes on each side to sear. Reduce heat to medium high and cook depending on thickness and desired degree of doneness.

4 Heat the marinade in a small saucepan or in the skillet used to cook the swordfish, until boiling for 1 minute.

5 Serve hot marinade over grilled fish with a pinch of fresh oregano for garnish.

PER SERVING: *Calories 395; Total fat: 27g; Saturated fat: 5 g; Cholesterol: 66 mg; Sodium: 294 mg; Carbohydrates: 3g; Fiber: 0g; Sugar: 1g; Protein: 34g.*

TIP: When grilling (or broiling), cook swordfish like you would a rare steak: Use high heat to sear the outside, and let it stay a little rare in the middle, about 5 minutes on one side, and then 2 to 3 minutes on the other for an inch-thick steak.

TIP: Serve with the Braised Broccoli Rabe and fresh lemon wedges.

Sautéed Branzino

PREP TIME: 10 MIN | **COOK TIME: 10 MIN** | **YIELD: 4 SERVINGS**

INGREDIENTS

¼ cup all-purpose flour

¼ cup extra-virgin olive oil

4 garlic cloves, peeled and roughly chopped

½ teaspoon crushed red pepper flakes

Four 6-ounce fillets branzino

½ cup dry white wine, such as Chardonnay

2 teaspoons fresh lemon juice

2 tablespoons fresh oregano

¼ teaspoon kosher salt

¼ teaspoon freshly ground black pepper

DIRECTIONS

1 Place the flour in a shallow dish. In a large skillet heat the olive oil over medium heat. Add the garlic and red pepper flakes and cook for 1 minute, but don't brown the garlic.

2 Flour both sides of the fish fillets and place them in the skillet, skin-side up. Cook for about 4 minutes.

3 Turn the fish, pour in the white wine, cover, and cook for 4 more minutes. Uncover and continue to cook for about 2 more minutes or until when a fork is twisted in the center of the fillet and the flesh separates easily.

4 Remove the fish to a platter. In the same skillet, turn the heat to medium high. Add the lemon juice, oregano, salt, and pepper. Scrape the pan with a wooden spoon and swirl the pan juices until slightly thickened. Pour the pan sauce over the fish.

PER SERVING: *Calories 432; Total fat: 25g; Saturated fat: 4 g; Cholesterol: 70 mg; Sodium: 231 mg; Carbohydrates: 13g; Fiber: 4g; Sugar: 1g; Protein: 37g.*

TIP: Branzino is a popular fish in the Mediterranean area. If it isn't available, substitute red snapper or Chilean seabass. The secret to delicious branzino, or any fish for that matter, is to not overcook. In general, for fully cooked pieces of fish, the general rule is 10 minutes total per inch of thickness of the fillet.

TIP: Serve with the Roasted Brussels Sprouts and some lemon wedges.

Making Mediterranean Side Dishes for Intermittent Fasting

The best way to make those anti-cancer, cruciferous veggies taste spectacular is to douse them with EVOO and roast or braise them. Cruciferous (comes from the Latin *cruciferae* meaning "cross bearing," because the four petals of this family resemble a cross) vegetables are a diverse group that pack a nutritional and inflammation-fighting one-two punch. Here is a list of common cruciferous veggies:

» Arugula

» Bok choy

» Broccoli

» Brussels sprouts

» Cabbage

» Cauliflower

» Collards

» Kale

» Radishes

» Watercress

Side dishes like the following recipes also help you follow another anti-inflammatory technique of eating, based on many budget-friendly, shelf-stable foods, like beans, lentils, nuts, seeds, and whole grains. Despite what you may have heard, potatoes, especially sweet potatoes, are true superfoods. Sweet potatoes are highly nutritious, a great source of fiber, vitamins, minerals, and disease-fighting antioxidants. When drizzled with EVOO and fresh rosemary and roasted to perfection, they become a candied naturally sweet side dish treat.

Roasted Cauliflower

PREP TIME: 30 MIN	COOK TIME: 25 MIN	YIELD: 4 SERVINGS

INGREDIENTS

2 tablespoons extra-virgin olive oil

2 Vidalia onions, peeled and quartered

6 garlic cloves, halved

4 cups cauliflower florets (approximately 1½ pounds)

Drizzle of extra virgin olive oil

1 tablespoon water

1 tablespoon Dijon mustard

½ teaspoon sea salt

¼ teaspoon freshly ground pepper

DIRECTIONS

1 Preheat oven to 475° F.

2 Heat the olive oil in a large skillet over medium heat. Add the onions and garlic; cook 5 minutes or until browned, stirring frequently. Remove from heat.

3 Place the cauliflower florets in a large mixing bowl. Combine the olive oil, water, and Dijon mustard and pour over the cauliflower, using your hands to coat the cauliflower with the liquid.

4 Mix the onion mixture and cauliflower together and spread on a roasting pan lined with parchment paper and coated with cooking spray. Sprinkle with salt and pepper.

5 Bake for 20 minutes or until golden brown, stirring occasionally.

PER SERVING: *Calories 110; Total fat: 7g; Saturated fat: 1g; Cholesterol: 0 mg; Sodium: 130mg; Carbohydrates: 10g; Fiber: 3g; Sugar: 4g; Protein: 3g.*

TIP: Spread the cauliflower out in an even layer so the florets aren't touching. Roasting on parchment paper will give your cauliflower a pan-fried finish.

Roasted Brussels Sprouts

PREP TIME: 5 MIN	COOK TIME: 35 MIN	YIELD: 4 SERVINGS

INGREDIENTS

1 pound Brussels sprouts, trimmed and cut in half

2 tablespoons extra-virgin olive oil

3 garlic cloves, peeled and sliced

½ teaspoon kosher salt

½ teaspoon freshly ground black pepper

DIRECTIONS

1 Preheat oven to 425° F.

2 In a glass baking dish, toss the Brussels sprouts with the olive oil, sliced garlic, salt, and pepper. Bake for 30 to 35 minutes until lightly browned.

PER SERVING: *Calories 113; Total fat: 7g; Saturated fat: 1g; Cholesterol: 0mg; Sodium: 174mg; Carbohydrates: 11g; Fiber: 4g; Sugar: 3g; Protein: 4g.*

TIP: To save time, buy the prewashed, bagged Brussels sprouts. When roasted with slices of fresh garlic, Brussels sprouts turn into a vegetable everyone will love.

Braised Broccoli Rabe

INGREDIENTS

4 quarts water

½ teaspoon kosher salt

2 bunches broccoli rabe

2 tablespoons extra-virgin olive oil

4 garlic cloves, peeled and chopped

¼ teaspoon crushed red pepper flakes

DIRECTIONS

1 In a large pot bring water and salt to a boil.

2 Trim and chop the broccoli rabe into 2-inch pieces. Drop the broccoli rabe in boiling water and cook for 3 minutes. Drain and cool in ice water for 30 minutes. Drain well.

3 In a large skillet heat the olive oil over medium-high heat. Add the garlic and red pepper flakes and cook until the garlic is golden brown. Add the broccoli rabe, cover, and lower the heat to medium low.

4 Cook for 4 minutes. Toss with salt to taste just before serving.

PER SERVING: *Calories 92; Total fat: 1g; Saturated fat: 1g; Cholesterol: 0mg; Sodium: 112mg; Carbohydrates: 5g; Fiber: 3g; Sugar: 1g; Protein: 4g.*

TIP: The secret to bright green broccoli rabe, without a hint of bitterness, is pre-cooking it in boiling water and cooling for up to 30 minutes in an ice-water bath.

Quinoa with Currants and Walnuts

PREP TIME: 25 MIN	COOK TIME: 20 MIN	YIELD: 6 SERVINGS

INGREDIENTS

1 cup quinoa, rinsed

2 cups reduced-sodium chicken or vegetable broth

¼ cup of dried currants

½ cup chopped walnuts, toasted

¼ cup sliced scallions (2 scallions)

DIRECTIONS

1 In a medium saucepan, bring the quinoa and broth to a boil. Cover, and reduce heat to low. Cook for 15 minutes.

2 After 5 minutes, open the lid and lightly fluff the quinoa with a fork to separate the grains. Gently stir in the currants, walnuts, and scallions. Serve warm or at room temperature.

PER SERVING: *Calories 194; Total fat: 8g; Saturated fat: 1.5g; Cholesterol: 0 mg; Sodium: 192mg; Carbohydrates: 26g; Fiber: 3g; Sugar: 4g; Protein: 7g.*

TIP: Rinse the quinoa in a fine-mesh strainer with cool running water before cooking to remove the *saponin,* a natural coating on the quinoa that can be an irritant to the stomach if not removed. Some quinoa is sold pre-rinsed.

Sweet Potato Steak Fries

PREP TIME: 5 MIN	COOK TIME: 40 MIN	YIELD: 4 SERVINGS

INGREDIENTS

4 sweet potatoes, large

2 tablespoons extra virgin olive oil

2 tablespoons fresh rosemary, minced

½ teaspoon salt

DIRECTIONS

1 Preheat the oven to 425° F. Spray a large cookie or baking sheet with olive oil nonstick spray.

2 Half the potatoes lengthwise and then continue to quarter them until they're steak fry wedge size. Toss the wedges with the oil, rosemary, and salt in a large bowl. Place the potatoes in a single layer on the baking pan with the skin side up.

3 Bake for about 20 minutes and then turn the potatoes so the opposite side is face up. Roast again until the potatoes are tender and golden-brown, 15 to 20 minutes more. Serve immediately.

PER SERVING: *Calories 170; Total fat: 7g; Saturated fat: 1.5g; Cholesterol: 0 mg; Sodium: 615mg; Carbohydrates: 26g; Fiber: 4g; Sugar: 5g; Protein: 2g.*

TIP: The addition of fresh rosemary and extra virgin olive oil give these sweet treat beta-carotene gold mines an extra antioxidant kick.

Diving into Desserts and Snacks for Intermittent Fasting

The beauty of intermittent fasting is that you can still eat the foods you love and stick to your healthy living program. The dessert recipes show you that eating desserts can also be nutritious. Many are made with sinfully divine dark chocolate. Now isn't this the best nutrition news to come along in decades? Dark chocolate — with a high content of cocoa — is now the new health food and a guilt-free superfood! The scientific evidence is stacking up linking consumption of deep, dark chocolate with phenomenal health benefits and especially for its salutary effect on your heart and blood vessels.

Flavonoids (the active ingredient in dark chocolate) work as potent antioxidants to protect you from *free radical damage,* the process which accelerates aging and promotes chronic illnesses such as heart disease and cancer. When choosing chocolate for health, the chocolate must be the flavonoid-rich dark variety because dark chocolate has a much higher percentage of cocoa than milk chocolate, and it's the cocoa that contains most of the flavonoids — plant substances that provide your body with a host of health benefits.

TIP

When concocting your own chocolate goodies, use natural unsweetened dark cocoa powder. If going for a bar, choose dark chocolate with at least 70 percent cocoa. Look at the ingredient list and make sure the first ingredient is cocoa or chocolate and not sugar. Also, avoid Dutch processed chocolate, chocolate that has been treated with a flavonoid-destroying alkalizing agent.

This section also includes a few recipes for snacks. Studies have shown that when making actual choices, people often make them unconsciously and more impulsively, meaning even though people often want to eat healthy, they sometimes just grab the junk food. Researchers found a substantial gap between healthy snack choice intentions and actual behavior. The best way to avoid reaching for the junk food is to clean out your kitchen and pantry and simply not keep the unhealthful snacks in the house.

Feel free to snack on foods during your eating windows. Just make sure that you grab nutritious snacks in lieu of empty-calorie junk foods. Here you can see that you can still munch on satisfying snacks that fulfill your impulses with these delicious and highly nutritious snacks.

Dark Chocolate Brownies with Walnuts

PREP TIME: 10 MIN	COOK TIME: 30 MIN	YIELD: 12 SERVINGS

INGREDIENTS

½ cup extra-virgin olive oil

2 teaspoons vanilla extract

½ cup Splenda sugar baking blend

½ cup Splenda brown sugar blend

2 whole eggs

¼ cup egg substitute

½ cup dark chocolate unsweetened cacao powder

½ cup all-purpose flour

½ cup dark chocolate chips

½ cup chopped walnuts

Pinch of salt

DIRECTIONS

1 Preheat the oven to 350° F. Line an 8x8 square baking pan with parchment paper.

2 Use a large mixing bowl to combine the olive oil, vanilla extract, sugar baking blend, and brown sugar blend. Mix with a fork or whisk until an even consistency is reached.

3 In a separate bowl, whisk the whole eggs and egg substitute with a fork for about 30 seconds.

4 In another separate bowl, combine cacao powder, flour, chocolate chips, walnuts, and pinch of salt. Pour in the eggs to the sugar mixture and stir a few times with a fork. Add the dry mixture in stages using a spoon or spatula. Gently fold the dry mixture into the wet mixture until even.

5 Transfer batter to the parchment-lined baking tray. Bake for 28 to 30 minutes or until the center of the brownies comes out clean with a fork/toothpick test. Leave brownies to firm and cool before removing from pan. Slice into 12 pieces.

PER SERVING: *Calories 240; Total fat: 17g; Saturated fat: 4g; Cholesterol: 30mg; Sodium: 65mg; Carbohydrates: 21g; Fiber: 2g; Sugar: 13g; Protein: 4g.*

TIP: For brownie frosting, mix 1 tablespoon of cacao powder with 1 teaspoon of brown Splenda baking blend and 1 to 2 teaspoons of water.

Angel Food Cake Pops

PREP TIME: 20 MIN	COOK TIME: 0 MINS	YIELD: 20 SERVINGS

INGREDIENTS

½ cup cream cheese (⅓ less fat) (Neufchatel)

¼ cup powdered sugar

One 10-inch angel food cake

20 paper lollipop sticks

1 cup dark chocolate baking chips

Optional toppings: sliced almonds, chopped walnuts, granola, sprinkles

DIRECTIONS

1 In a large bowl, whisk together the cream cheese and powdered sugar. Break up the angel food cake into large pieces (about 6 cups).

2 Pulse in a food processor until fine crumbs form. Transfer crumbs to the cream cheese mixture and form a dough. Shape into 1-inch balls and insert lollipop sticks. Transfer cake pops to a large plate and freeze for about 20 minutes.

3 Place the dark chocolate chips into separate microwave-safe bowl. Heat for 30 seconds. Remove and stir until the chips are melted and smooth (you may need to microwave for another 20 seconds).

4 Remove the pops from the refrigerator and dip into the chocolate bowl; sprinkle with desired toppings. Place cake pops on a wax-covered plate/baking sheet. Place chocolate-covered cake pops into the refrigerator for 20 minutes or freeze overnight.

PER SERVING (1 POP, NO TOPPING): *Calories 131; Total fat: 7g; Saturated fat: 2g; Cholesterol: 13 mg; Sodium: 218mg; Carbohydrates: 26g; Fiber: 0g; Sugar: 15g; Protein: 2g.*

TIP: The cake balls need to be extremely cold before dipping. You can find lollipop sticks at craft stores.

Dark Chocolate–Dipped Strawberries

PREP TIME: 15 MIN	COOK TIME: 10 MIN	YIELD: 12 SERVINGS

INGREDIENTS

1½ cup 72 percent cacao dark chocolate premium baking chips

12 fresh strawberries, large

Optional toppings: chopped pistachios or walnuts

DIRECTIONS

1 Wash and dry the strawberries.

2 Fill the bottom of a double boiler with water and set on low heat. Place the chocolate chips in the top of the double boiler over hot water (not boiling water) and let the chocolate melt. Don't cover the pot. Stir constantly until the chocolate melts and is smooth. Remove the top of the boiler from the hot water.

3 Put the chocolate chips in a glass bowl and place the bowl on the hot water in the saucepan. Stir constantly and let the chocolate melt. Carefully remove from the glass bowl from the saucepan; it will be hot.

4 Hold one strawberry by the stem and dip it into the chocolate until it's about three-quarters covered. Then dip the chocolate-covered strawberry in a topping. Place the chocolate-covered strawberry on a baking sheet lined with parchment paper to harden. Repeat with other strawberries.

PER SERVING: *Calories 76; Total fat: 5g; Saturated fat: 1g; Cholesterol: 1mg; Sodium: 5mg; Carbohydrates:4g; Fiber: 1g; Sugar: 2g; Protein: 0g.*

TIP: It takes around 20 to 30 minutes for the chocolate to harden. Be sure to use a high-quality brand of baking chocolate chips. High quality baking chocolate chips taste less processed, melt easier, and help give the strawberries a nice beautiful coat after dipping.

TIP: If you don't have double boiler, fill the saucepan half full with water and place it on low heat.

European Hot Chocolate

INGREDIENTS

1½ cups milk, 1 percent

½ cup soy creamer

1 packet Splenda or stevia

1 teaspoon instant coffee

½ bar of 72 percent chocolate bar, 8.8 oz

Dollop of fat-free whipped topping

DIRECTIONS

1 In a medium saucepan over medium heat, whisk together the milk, creamer, sweetener, and instant coffee until small bubbles form around the edges. Don't boil. Chop the chocolate bar into small pieces and add to saucepan.

2 Stir saucepan mixture for about 5 minutes to melt or until desired consistency is reached. Serve in an espresso cup and top with fat-free whipped cream.

PER SERVING: *Calories 230; Total fat: 15g; Saturated fat: 1g; Cholesterol: 1mg; Sodium: 35mg; Carbohydrates: 18g; Fiber: 0g; Sugar: <1g; Protein: 4g.*

TIP: Serve in espresso cups for a ¼-cup serving size. This recipe is very rich and satisfying even at a small serving size.

Frozen Date Bars

| PREP TIME: 20 MIN | COOK TIME: 3 HOURS | YIELD: 24 SERVINGS |

INGREDIENTS

1 cup of old-fashioned rolled oats

¼ cup of pumpkin seeds

¼ cup of flax seeds

¼ cup of chia seeds

¼ cup of sunflower seeds

¼ cup of ground walnuts

¼ teaspoon kosher salt

¼ teaspoon pepper

¼ cup of extra virgin olive oil

10 Medjool dates

Unsweetened coconut flakes (optional)

DIRECTIONS

1 Mix the oats, seeds, walnuts, salt, and pepper together. Add the oil and stir until the seeds, nuts, and oats become thoroughly mixed.

2 Preheat oven to 350° F. Line a baking sheet with parchment paper and spread oat/nut/seed mixture onto the sheet evenly. Cook granola in the oven for 15 minutes or until it reaches a golden hue. Toss the granola halfway through for an even toast. After the granola bakes, remove from the oven and let it cool for at least 30 minutes.

3 Pit the dates and transfer to a food processor. Blend into a paste. In a large mixing bowl, add date paste and mix in cooled granola. Using either a mixing spoon or your hands, mash the granola into the dates to create a consistent, sticky mixture.

4 Line a baking dish with a sheet of parchment paper and spread granola mixture evenly onto the dish. If you want, add coconut flakes as topping.

5 Freeze for 1 hour. Take the tray out and cut bars. Put the bars back into the freezer until completely solid.

PER SERVING: *Calories 100; Total fat: 6g; Saturated fat: 1g; Cholesterol: 0 mg; Sodium: 45mg; Carbohydrates: 11g; Fiber: 3g; Sugar: 6g; Protein: 2g.*

TIP: Hand-mixing granola with dates is the best way to evenly mix all ingredients, but it does get messy and oily on your hands.

TIP: Store the bars in the freezer; they'll melt and crumble if left out at room temperature.

Berry Citrus Yogurt Parfait

PREP TIME: 10 MIN	COOK TIME: 0 MIN	YIELD: 4 SERVINGS

INGREDIENTS

1 pint nonfat Greek yogurt

5 pieces crystallized ginger, chopped

⅓ cup orange clover honey plus an extra drizzle

Zest from 1 orange

2 pints fresh blackberries

DIRECTIONS

1 In a medium bowl, combine the yogurt, ginger, honey, and orange zest. Divide the blackberries among 4 dessert parfait dishes. Top each parfait with ¼ of the yogurt mixture. Drizzle each with honey and serve.

PER SERVING: *Calories 250; Total fat: 0.5g; Saturated fat: 0g; Cholesterol: 5mg; Sodium: 45mg; Carbohydrates:508g; Fiber: 7g; Sugar: 39g; Protein: 14g.*

TIP: Add a dash of ground ginger spice for extra ginger flavor.

Pumpkin Pie Greek Yogurt

PREP TIME: 5 MIN	COOK TIME: 0 MIN	YIELD: 1 SERVING

INGREDIENTS

6-ounce container fat-free Greek yogurt

¼ cup canned pumpkin (no additives)

1 tablespoon orange clover honey or 2 packets Splenda

¼ teaspoon pumpkin pie spice

2 tablespoons fat-free whipped topping

1 tablespoon walnuts, diced

DIRECTIONS

1 In a medium bowl, combine the yogurt, pumpkin, sweetener of choice, and pumpkin pie spice. Place yogurt in a parfait glass, top with a dollop of whipped topping, and sprinkle with walnuts.

PER SERVING: *Calories 170; Total fat: 5g; Saturated fat: 0g; Cholesterol: 0 mg; Sodium: 70 mg; Carbohydrates:16g; Fiber: 3g; Sugar: 10g; Protein: 17g.*

TIP: Greek yogurt contains nearly triple the amount of protein as regular yogurt, due to the straining process, which results in a thicker consistency.

Chapter **22**

Creating Your 5:2 Intermittent Fasting Recipes

RECIPES IN THIS CHAPTER

Cajun Grilled Chicken

Honey-Crusted Salmon with Spinach

⏱ **Farro Salad**

⏱ **Cheesy Bean Burrito**

⏱ **Whole Grain Linguini with Cannellini Beans**

⏱ **Avocado Hummus Sandwich**

Whole Grain Linguini with Clams

Bean and Turkey Slow Cooker Chili

Sweet Pomegranate Chicken with Couscous

Chocolate Berry Protein Smoothie

I f you chose to follow the 5:2 intermittent fasting plan, then you're choosing two days a week (not consecutive) where you'll restrict your calories. There is no rule for what or when to eat on fasting days — just that the calories are controlled.

The idea of eating only 500 or 600 calories a day is intimidating. The good news is you don't have to starve on those fasting days. The trick is to drink lots of calorie-free liquids, and when it's time to eat, fill up on highly nutritious meals that contain a nice amount of protein and fiber (both are filling) and get the nutrition you need from healthy fats, fruit, and vegetables.

The recipes in this chapter are easy to prepare and portion controlled — the first section for 500-calorie meals for women and the second section for 600-calorie meals for men. By cooking these meals, you can master portion control. During the past 20 years portion sizes have gotten larger, which is a likely contributing factor to the ever-expanding American waistline. In fact, some food items have more than doubled in size, adding additional calories to your plate and unwanted pounds to your body.

On your 5:2 intermittent fasting days, tame the hunger by having a plan. Have your meal at a time when you're confident you can make it the rest of the day without eating. Chapter 12 provides more information about the 5:2 intermittent fasting plan.

Making 500-Calorie Meals for Women

If you're eating just 500 calories, you need to make every bite count. In the following recipes, you can see that adding in lots of nonstarchy, super low-calorie vegetables can help you stretch your food intake. You may also want to start these days with a meal of a heaping leafy green salad to stave off hunger (make sure you're very judicious with the dressing). If you prefer to space out your 500 calories, feel free. Just remember to use a calculator and do the calorie calcs, journaling your eating to ensure you stay within the 500 calories.

Keep motivated on your fasting days with the notion that you can do anything in a day. Yes, 500 calories is a small meal, but you can do it with that knowledge that tomorrow you can eat normally!

Here are several tips to keep you on track during your fasting days:

>> **Drink plenty of calorie-free fluids.** Your fasting days are when you really want to drink up those liquids; doing so will help fill your stomach and take your mind off hunger.

>> **Count your calories.** This type of intermittent fasting plan is composed of two days per week where you really do need to calculate those calories. Weighing and measuring foods is always helpful.

>> **Flavor your foods.** Because every bite counts, make sure you eat slowly and savor every bite of highly flavorful foods.

>> **Eat highly nutritious meals with protein.** Protein is the most satiating of the three macronutrients (carbs, fat, and protein). Try eating a few egg whites before your meal — pure protein with negligible calories.

Cajun Grilled Chicken

PREP TIME: 30 MIN | COOK TIME: 15 MIN | YIELD: 2 SERVINGS

INGREDIENTS

½ teaspoon dried oregano

½ teaspoon dried thyme

1 teaspoon smoked or regular paprika

¼ teaspoon cayenne pepper

1 garlic clove, finely chopped

1 teaspoon canola oil

Four 5-ounce skinless, boneless chicken breasts

Bean salad

2 tomatoes, diced

⅔ cup frozen sweet corn, defrosted

1 cup canned black-eyed or cannellini beans, rinsed and drained

2 scallions, chopped

¼ cup sundried tomatoes

Zest and juice of 1 lime

1 tablespoon fresh cilantro leaves, chopped

Guacamole

1 ripe avocado

¼ teaspoon red chili pepper

½ tablespoon extra-virgin olive oil

1 lime, juiced

1 tablespoon fresh cilantro leaves, chopped

DIRECTIONS

1 For the chicken seasoning, mix all the herbs, spices, finely chopped garlic clove, and oil in a large plastic bag, add water to make the marinade more liquid. Place a chicken breast between two sheets of waxed parchment or clear plastic film. Pound with a mallet or rolling pin to flatten; transfer to the plastic bag and repeat with remaining breasts. Mix adequately and seal. Set aside bag to marinate for 15 minutes.

2 For the bean salad, de-seed and dice the tomatoes. Add to a large mixing bowl with the corn, beans, chopped scallions, finely chopped sundried tomatoes, and cilantro. Zest the lime and then cut in half. Add the zest and juice of the lime and mix thoroughly into the salad.

3 For the guacamole, scoop and pit 1 whole avocado and mash to preferred consistency. Add finely chopped chili pepper, olive oil, lime juice, and cilantro. Mix in by mashing with a fork.

4 Lightly grease grill surface and preheat grill to medium-high heat. Place chicken on the grill for 7 to 8 minutes. Flip over and cook an additional 7 to 8 minutes or until no pink remains and chicken reaches 165 degrees F. Serve each chicken breast on a plate with the bean salad and a scoop of guacamole.

PER SERVING: *Calories 520; Total fat: 23g; Saturated fat: 3.5g; Cholesterol: 80mg; Sodium: 150mg; Carbohydrates: 42g; Fiber: 16g; Sugar: 10g; Protein: 45g.*

Honey-Crusted Salmon with Spinach

PREP TIME: 10 MIN	COOK TIME: 15 MIN	YIELD: 4 SERVINGS

INGREDIENTS

1½ tablespoons Dijon mustard

1½ tablespoons honey

2 garlic cloves, minced

¾ cup Panko breadcrumbs

2 tablespoons chopped fresh parsley

1 teaspoon lemon zest

1 tablespoon extra-virgin olive oil

Four 6-ounce skinless salmon fillets

Freshly ground black pepper

Sea salt, optional

2 tablespoons extra-virgin olive oil

6 cloves garlic minced

6 cups fresh baby spinach

½ teaspoon kosher salt

¼ teaspoon freshly grated black pepper

Lemon slices for garnish

DIRECTIONS

1 Preheat the oven to 400 degrees F. Spray a large baking dish with nonstick olive oil cooking spray.

2 In a small bowl whisk together the Dijon mustard, honey, and garlic. In another bowl, mix the breadcrumbs, parsley, and lemon zest. Then drizzle in the olive oil to the bread crumb mixture and mix. Brush the top of each salmon fillet with the honey mixture and then dip in the bread crumb mixture to coat. Put salmon fillets in a single layer on a baking dish in the oven and cook for about 15 minutes until the salmon is cooked through.

3 While the salmon is baking, prepare the spinach. Heat oil over medium-high heat in a fry pan. Add the garlic and cook for 1 min.

4 Add spinach, kosher salt, and black pepper. Toss the spinach for 1 to 2 minutes until mostly wilted.

5 Remove from heat and serve with salmon with lemon wedges on the side.

PER SERVING: *Calories 500; Total fat: 28g; Saturated fat: 7 g; Cholesterol: 85 mg; Sodium: 370 mg; Carbohydrates: 22g; Fiber: 2g; Sugar: 6g; Protein: 37g.*

TIP: Salmon is such an easy fish to prepare, tastes great and is super nutritious. Salmon is low in mercury and packed with healthy omega-3 fat. Buy wild over farmed, if available.

Farro Salad

PREP TIME: 10 MIN	COOK TIME: 20 MIN	YIELD: 4 SERVINGS

INGREDIENTS

4 tablespoon extra-virgin olive oil, divided

2 cups whole farro, rinsed

6 cups water

4 cups organic baby arugula

4 tablespoons fresh dill, chopped

1 cup frozen peas, thawed

4 ounces feta cheese, crumbled

Dressing

3 tablespoons fresh lemon juice

1 teaspoon lemon zest

DIRECTIONS

1 Place 1 tablespoon of the olive oil in a medium saucepan over medium heat. Allow olive oil to simmer in pan. Add the farro to simmering olive oil and stir until fragrant for about 3 minutes.

2 Add water and dash of salt. Bring water to a boil, cover, and reduce heat to low. Allow to simmer for about 35 minutes or until the farro is tender and chewy (al dente).

3 Drain the farro using a fine-mesh sieve. Spread across a rimmed baking sheet to cool at room temperature.

4 Use a large serving bowl to make salad dressing. Whisk together the 3 remaining tablespoons of olive oil, 3 tablespoons of lemon juice, 1 teaspoon of lemon zest, ½ teaspoon of salt, and ¼ teaspoon of pepper. Set aside.

5 In a large serving bowl, add the arugula, farro, dill, and peas. Toss the ingredients and sprinkle with feta and pour in the dressing.

PER SERVING: *Calories 500; Total fat: 19g; Saturated fat: 5g; Cholesterol: 10mg; Sodium: 590mg; Carbohydrates: 69g; Fiber: 8g; Sugar: 3g; Protein: 20g.*

TIP: Farro is an extremely nutritious ancient grain. Grocery stores typically sell three types of farro: pearled, semi-pearled, and whole. Be sure to buy the whole version.

Cheesy Bean Burrito

PREP TIME: 15 MIN	COOK TIME: 5 MIN	YIELD: 1 SERVINGS

INGREDIENTS

2 teaspoons extra-virgin olive oil

1 clove garlic, chopped

½ small onion, sliced thin

4 ounces (about ¼ of a can black beans, rinsed and drained)

½ red bell pepper, chopped

2 tablespoons sweet corn kernels, frozen

1 plum tomato, chopped into small pieces

¼ cup shredded cheddar jack cheese, reduced fat

One 10-inch flour tortilla

¼ cup fresh salsa

DIRECTIONS

1 In a large skillet, add the olive oil, garlic, and onion, and sauté over medium–high heat until onion is translucent and is lightly browned. Add the beans, red pepper, corn, and tomato, and heat until mixture has warmed and corn has defrosted (about 5 minutes), stirring occasionally.

2 To make the burrito, take one large flour tortilla, add the bean mixture, and top with shredded cheese. Roll the tortilla and heat in the microwave for 30 seconds until cheese has melted. Top with salsa and serve.

PER SERVING: *Calories 480; Total fat: 16g; Saturated fat: 4.5g; Cholesterol: 5mg; Sodium: 940mg; Carbohydrates: 72g; Fiber: 10g; Sugar: 11g; Protein: 17g.*

TIP: Use a fruit salsa, such as mango, to add extra flavor and nutrients.

Whole Grain Linguini with Cannellini Beans

PREP TIME: 10 MIN	COOK TIME: 15 MIN	YIELD: 4 SERVINGS

INGREDIENTS

8 ounces whole-grain linguini

2 tablespoons extra-virgin olive oil

One 14.5-ounce can petite diced tomatoes

One 15-ounce can cannellini beans, rinsed and drained

3 tablespoons jarred pesto sauce

3 tablespoons capers

1 tablespoon shredded Parmesan cheese

DIRECTIONS

1 Cook the pasta according to directions; drain and set aside in a large pasta bowl.

2 In a large skillet, heat the olive oil over medium heat. Add the diced tomatoes and beans and simmer for about 5 minutes until heated. Stir in the pesto and heat for another few minutes.

3 Stir in the capers and remove from the heat. Add the sauce to pasta, tossing gently to coat. Top with grated Parmesan if desired.

PER SERVING: *Calories 470; Total fat: 25g; Saturated fat: 2.5g; Cholesterol: 0mg; Sodium: 900mg; Carbohydrates: 70g; Fiber: 7g; Sugar: 4g; Protein: 17g.*

TIP: Rinse the beans several times with water to eliminate much of the excessive sodium typically added to canned beans.

Creating 600-Calorie Meals for Men

What does 600 calories of food look like? Depending on your food choices, it may not look like much. However, you can stretch out those calories by adding in lots of low-calorie foods. This section includes some full 600 calorie nutritious meal recipes. They're composed of lean protein, healthy fats, fiber, vitamins, minerals, and antioxidants.

Eating one meal a day may not be the best strategy for you. Some people function best by beginning the day with a small breakfast, whereas others find it best to start eating as late as possible. Because calorie intake is strictly limited to 600 calories for men, it makes sense to use your calorie budget wisely. Try to focus on nutritious, high-fiber, high-protein foods that will make you feel full without consuming too many calories.

TIP

For five days per week, you eat normally and don't have to think about restricting calories. That doesn't mean you can go hog wild on your eating days as a reward. If you try to make up for lost calories from your fasting days on your normal eating days, you'll lose out on the miraculous health benefits of intermittent fasting.

Here are a few examples of foods that work well for fasting days:

>> Soups

>> Generous portions of non-starchy vegetables

>> Non-fat yogurt with berries

>> Egg whites

>> Cauliflower rice

Triple Decker Hummus Sandwich

PREP TIME: 10 MIN | COOK TIME: 0 MIN | YIELD: 1 SERVING

INGREDIENTS

3 slices whole grain or rye toast

1 tablespoon pesto

2 tablespoons hummus

1 cup baby arugula, organic

1 pitted avocado

½ teaspoon pepper

8 cherry tomatoes

DIRECTIONS

1 Toast three slices of whole grain or rye bread.

2 Mix pesto with hummus and then spread 1 tablespoon of pesto hummus onto each slice of bread.

3 Scoop out the avocado and slice. Sprinkle ½ teaspoon of pepper on top of the avocado for seasoning.

4 Slice the cherry tomatoes in flat halves.

5 Make your sandwich: layer bread, then hummus, then arugula, avocado, and tomato. Repeat then top with last slice of bread, hummus side down. Cut in half for easier eating.

PER SERVING: *Calories 590; Total fat: 37g; Saturated fat: 7g; Cholesterol: 60mg; Sodium: 610mg; Carbohydrates: 61g; Fiber: 18g; Sugar: 6g; Protein: 17g.*

TIP: Adding the arugula layer directly on top of the hummus and before adding the avocado helps to keep the ingredients in place. For extra flavor, add a squeeze of lemon juice on top of the hummus.

Whole Grain Linguini with Clams

PREP TIME: 10 MIN	COOK TIME: 20 MIN	YIELD: 4 SERVINGS

INGREDIENTS

12 ounces whole grain linguini, uncooked

2 tablespoons extra-virgin olive oil

4 cloves garlic, sliced thinly

½ teaspoon crushed red pepper flakes

¼ cup dry white wine, preferably Sauvignon Blanc

Two 6.5-ounce cans minced clams, drained (with liquid from cans reserved)

¼ cup fresh parsley, chopped

1 tablespoon fresh basil, chopped

4 tablespoons Parmesan cheese

DIRECTIONS

1 Cook the linguini according to the instructions on the package until it's al dente, and then drain it well. Before draining, put ½ cup pasta liquid aside.

2 In a large skillet, gently heat the oil over medium–low heat. Add the garlic and red pepper flakes and cook, stirring constantly, for about 15 to 20 seconds, until fragrant.

3 Add the reserved clam juice, white wine, and reserved pasta water to the skillet. Reduce the heat to low and simmer gently until the liquid begins to reduce, about 1 minute.

4 Add the clams and simmer until just heated, about 30 to 60 seconds. Then stir in the parsley and basil.

5 Add the pasta and toss until it's well coated, about 30 to 45 seconds. Top with the grated Parmesan cheese, and serve immediately.

PER SERVING: *Calories 580; Total fat: 14 g; Saturated fat: 3 g; Cholesterol: 80 mg; Sodium: 240 mg; Carbohydrates: 68 g; Fiber: 1g; Sugar: 3 g; Protein: 50g.*

TIP: The salt used to preserve inexpensive cooking wine makes it unpotable. Better to use a real Sauvignon Blanc.

Bean and Turkey Slow Cooker Chili

PREP TIME: 10 MIN	COOK TIME: 4 HRS	YIELD: 4 SERVINGS

INGREDIENTS

1 tablespoon extra-virgin olive oil

1¼ pounds extra lean ground turkey breast

½ medium onion, chopped

Two 28-ounce can no-salt-added crushed tomatoes

Two 16-ounce cans dark red kidney beans, rinsed and drained

One 15-ounce can black beans, rinsed and drained

2 tablespoons chili powder

1 teaspoon red pepper flakes

½ tablespoon garlic power

½ tablespoon ground cumin

1 pinch ground black pepper

1 pinch ground allspice

Salt to taste, optional

DIRECTIONS

1 Heat the oil in a large skillet over medium–high heat.

2 Place the turkey and onions in the skillet and cook until evenly browned, about 5 minutes.

3 Coat the inside of a slow cooker with nonstick spray.

4 Mix together the turkey, crushed tomatoes, kidney beans, black beans, and onion. Season with the chili powder, red pepper flakes, garlic powder, cumin, black pepper, and allspice and blend.

5 Cover and cook 4 hours on high. Serve hot. Add salt to taste.

PER SERVING: *Calories 630; Total fat: 7g; Saturated fat: 1 g; Cholesterol: 70 mg; Sodium: 740 mg; Carbohydrates: 84g; Fiber: 12 g; Sugar: 15g; Protein: 60g.*

TIP: Serve warm, garnished with a touch of fat-free shredded cheddar cheese for flavor. If you have the time, cook the chili on low heat for 8 hours. Simmering recipes over longer periods of time extracts all those subtle flavors.

Sweet Pomegranate Chicken with Couscous

PREP TIME: 10 MIN	COOK TIME: 15 MIN	YIELD: 4 SERVINGS

INGREDIENTS

2 tablespoons extra-virgin olive oil

1 large red onion, halved and thinly sliced

1 chicken bouillon cube

Four 5-ounce chicken breasts

2 tablespoons harissa

¾ cup pomegranate juice

½ cup pomegranate seeds

1 cup couscous, preferably whole wheat

Dash ground black pepper

Dash salt ½ cup toasted almond pieces

¼ cup mint, chopped

DIRECTIONS

1 Heat the oil in a large skillet on medium heat. Add the red onions and stir. Crumble the chicken bouillon cube by hand and add to the cooking pan with onions. Cook for several minutes, allowing the onions to soften.

2 Push the onions to one side of the pan and add the chicken breasts until they brown on the sides. Flip the chicken and stir in the harissa and pomegranate juice. Let simmer for 10 minutes, until the sauce thickens and chicken is cooked through. Stir in ¼ cup of pomegranate seeds.

3 To make the couscous, boil 1¼ cups water in a kettle or small pot. In a large bowl, add dry couscous with a pinch of salt and pepper. Pour enough boiling water to cover the couscous. Cover the bowl with a towel and set aside for 5 minutes.

4 After 5 minutes, fluff the couscous with a fork and stir in the almonds and mint.

5 Serve the chicken and sauce on top of the couscous mixture, and sprinkle remaining ¼ cup pomegranate seeds on top.

PER SERVING: *Calories 590; Total fat: 23g; Saturated fat: 2g; Cholesterol: 80mg; Sodium: 360mg; Carbohydrates: 54g; Fiber: 1g; Sugar: 15g; Protein: 45g.*

TIP: To avoid excess sugar intake, be sure to use a pomegranate juice with no sugar added.

Chocolate Berry Protein Smoothie

PREP TIME: 5 MIN	COOK TIME: NONE	YIELD: 1 SERVING

INGREDIENTS

12 fluid ounces unsweetened vanilla almond milk

1 tablespoon peanut butter (can substitute with any nut/seed butter)

1 tablespoon chia seeds

½ fresh banana

¼ cup frozen wild blueberries

1 scoop vegan chocolate protein powder

DIRECTIONS

1 Place ingredients in a blender in the order listed. Blend until smooth and serve.

PER SERVING: *Calories 600; Total fat: 19g; Saturated fat: 2g; Cholesterol: 0 mg; Sodium: 780mg; Carbohydrates: 48g; Fiber: 8g; Sugar: 20g; Protein: 61g.*

TIP: For extra nutrition and negligible extra calories, add in 3 ounces frozen organic spinach.

6

Using Tools for Success

Discover the tools you need to stick to your intermittent fasting plan of choice.

Incorporate the skills to sustain your new lifestyle over the long term.

Tap into the available resources and support to keep you motivated and on track.

Chapter **23**

Tracking Your Intermittent Fasting Progress

U tilizing goal-setting tips to ensure you stay on the right track, journaling, and graphing your results are all great success strategies. This chapter gives you all the tools you need to start in your intermittent fasting toolbox. Studies have shown without any shadow of a doubt, that people who are most successful at making and sustaining positive lifestyle behavior changes track what they eat, how much exercise they do, and what they weigh over time.

Plenty of tools in your toolbox can aid you in navigating through your fasting journey. Chapter 2 emphasizes the importance of goal setting. In the following sections, I focus on the importance of using a journal to record your goals. In fact, a journal to write down how you are feeling and what positive and negative experiences you're having is probably the best tool to lead you to reaching your goals.

Journaling for Success

Many people who follow a version of intermittent fasting not only lose body fat but they also report having more mental clarity, more energy for vigorous work-outs, better sleep, and relief from digestive issues. Journaling and memorializing these symptoms will allow you to look back on your journey. When you hit the inevitable rough patch, you can look back at the positive experiences that you journaled about to keep going. Journaling your thoughts, experiences, and goals during your intermittent fasting journey is so valuable because it:

>> **Clarifies your goals.** Having set goals that you've created for yourself frees your mind to focus your efforts and use your time and resources productively. Every day make sure you do something towards your goal, no matter how small that action may seem and write it down.

>> **Develops motivation.** The act of recording your intermittent fasting experi-ences is extremely helpful in keeping you motivated. You'll have created a little sanctuary of inspiration in your journal. Refer to it often and put it to good use as a positive tool to reflect your inner strength.

>> **Helps you visualize success.** If you stick to your intermittent fasting day but have no record of it, how can you remember that you actually did it? By having something to see, in black and white, such as a reduction in your waist size, you'll grasp the tremendous benefits you're gaining from your hard work and lifestyle change.

>> **Rewards successes.** One of the most important behavior modification tools at your disposal is recognizing small successes and giving yourself a reward (nonfood related, of course!). Celebrating your successes, no matter how small, is another way to keep you motivated.

Use a tracking strategy that works for you. If you prefer to put pen to paper and write down everything you experience, then carry a small accountability journal with you. It doesn't have to be a set journal style; you can even simply jot down a one word positive step you took toward your goals on your daily calendar.

However, if logging on to a computer or using your smart phone works for you, then use what works for you. The kind of tracking tool — paper, computer, or mobile phone — isn't important. What's important is you consistently record your experiences.

By journaling, you have a powerful tool that provides insight into your personal behaviors. This tool enables you to reflect on and discover how to improve your overall eating patterns. For example, ask yourself these questions: Did a certain food or situation cause you to eat too much at that meal? Was it a good week or a not-so-good week in terms of sticking to your healthy lifestyle behaviors? What were the circumstances that led to the week's positive or negative results?

If the thought of making such drastic changes to your lifestyle is overwhelming, remember, you are in control and you choose the plan that will work for you. Take one day at a time. Changing behavior is a difficult task because despite the best laid plans, life often gets in the way of perfection, so, don't be too hard on yourself. Aim for getting a B in your intermittent fasting program and not an A. Take small steps with the knowledge that the minute you start somewhere, you'll be making a positive lifestyle change, putting you on the road to a healthier and happier life.

Graphing Your Progress

If one of your long-term goals is losing weight and body fat, then graphing is a marvelous tool for helping to make it happen. Take the assessment tools from Chapter 2 where you set your goals and graph your numbers over time in your body composition graph. You can graph your body weight weekly and/or your percent body fat and/or your waist measurements in three-month time frames.

Whether you weigh in once a week or month, knowing how close you are to reaching a weight-loss goal and reflecting on how far you have come is highly motivating. Creating a graph gives you a visual picture of weight and body fat fluctuations over time, allowing you to identify if there are patterns or plateaus in your weight loss. A graph can show you your accomplishments and motivate you to reach your goal weight and maintain it after you get there. Numbers don't lie and looking at the numbers for your goals on a regular basis will keep you heading in the right direction.

People don't maintain an exact weight their entire lives. The object is to attain and remain within your personal healthy weight range in the years to come. Here are some helpful graphing guidelines:

>> **Time your measurements.** Record your body weight on a weekly basis (if you're okay with weighing), your waist girth, and your percentage of body fat every four weeks.

>> **Analyze body composition changes.** Compare the differences in your weight, waist measurement, and percentage of body fat over time to determine if changes observed in weight are due to fat loss, muscle gain, or hydration level. For example, you may notice an increase in your weight; however, it may be due to an increase in your muscle mass rather than a gain

in body fat. On the other hand, if you lost a noticeable amount of weight on the scale but not your percentage of body fat, the weight loss may be due to a loss of muscle mass or water instead of fat.

>> **Become accountable to yourself.** Record your measurements and note the time of year and your exercise habits and proceed to analyze the peaks and valleys. What was happening in your life when you were at your fighting weight? What happened to your intermittent fasting healthy lifestyle behaviors when you packed on a few pounds?

WARNING

Remember that your body weight is *not* the only indicator of your health and wellness. Pay attention to your energy levels and your medical assessments. If you're eating healthfully, exercising, and following your intermittent fasting protocol, more than likely your body is becoming healthier even if your weight doesn't change by a significant amount.

Consider this example: Mike graphed 12 weeks of his intermittent fasting program. Mike is 40 years old, 5-10, and 210 pounds when he started. His body fat percentage is 30 percent, a BMI of 30 (considered obese), and his waist circumference is 40 inches. Mike was athletic but had gained weight around his middle since college. His goals were to lose weight and body fat, especially whittling away the dangerous belly fat that had increased his risk of cardiovascular disease. He started the Eat-Stop-Eat intermittent fast (which I discuss in Chapter 13), choosing to perform a 24-hour fast once a week, combined with a plant-based Mediterranean diet and his regular exercise routine (daily cardio and weight training three times a week). As you can see in Figure 23-1, Mike lost 30 pounds, 6 percent body fat, and 5 inches off his waist in those 12 weeks.

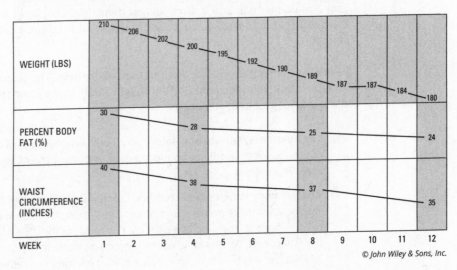

FIGURE 23-1: Mike's sample body composition graph.

© John Wiley & Sons, Inc.

You can keep track of your own body composition changes during your personal intermittent fasting journey with Figure 23-2. Make copies and fill in the shaded areas.

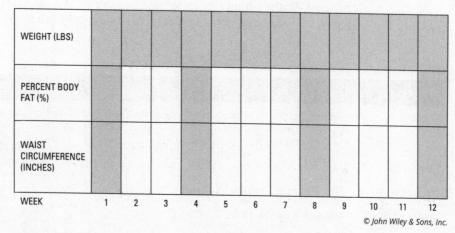

FIGURE 23-2: Weight, body fat, and waist circumference body composition graph.

© John Wiley & Sons, Inc.

Monitoring your SMART goals

Chapter 2 helps you create your first SMART goal for the week. Now what? Every day refresh your memory what your SMART goal is. Ask yourself if you're on the path to accomplishing your goal. If you're having a problem accomplishing your goal, determine why, take appropriate action, and change the goal to make it attainable and realistic. Celebrating success and reinforcing the importance of having achieved a goal, no matter how small is essential. Monitoring your SMART goal progress means you clarify your thoughts, focus your efforts, use your time productively, increase your motivation, and improve your chances of achieving what you want out of your intermittent fast.

TIP

One easy and highly motivating tool is to create a one-week calendar (starting with tomorrow) with the days of the week and actual dates. Depending on what intermittent fasting plan you choose, pick a single day and write down exactly what you'll eat or drink in those 24 hours. For example, if you're following the Eat-Stop-Eat program, choose either one or two nonconsecutive days per week during which you'll completely abstain from eating — or fast — for a full 24-hour period. During the 24-hour fast, you can't consume anything except for calorie-free drinks. If you're doing one day (instead of two), say a Tuesday, put your calendar somewhere in sight and pencil in exactly what you'll be consuming for those 24 hours — for example: 32 ounces of lemon water, two cups of green tea, and one cup of chamomile herbal tea with one packet of stevia. By setting a goal of just one day, you can focus and accomplish just about anything you set your mind to!

To make sure your goals are clear and reachable, make sure your goals are SMART goals. Table 23-1 gives you an example of Jenna's first weekly SMART goal worksheet. Jenna is following the Eat–Stop–Eat style of intermittent fasting. Because she just started, she wants to ensure that she is successful in achieving her goal, so she's fully committed and knows that she can accomplish her goal. Figure 23-3 shows an example of the way Jenna keeps track and motivates herself.

TABLE 23-1 **Jenna's SMART Goals for Week 1**

SMART	Goal
Specific	Drink 24 ounces of water, black coffee as desired, and two cups of calorie-free organic cinnamon herbal tea (sweetened with 1 packet of stevia) and consume nothing from Monday night to Wednesday morning.
Measurable	Measure the water in a measuring cup and transfer it to my water bottle.
Attainable	I know I can do anything in a single day.
Realistic	This goal is doable for me to accomplish.
Time-bound	Start drinking my fluids when I wake up Tuesday morning (8 a.m.) until before bed Tuesday night. At 6 p.m. drink my two cups of cinnamon tea.

Sunday	Monday	Tuesday	Wednesday	Thursday	Friday	Saturday
Normal Eating	Normal Eating	Today is the day! FIT or fasting, Intermittent Tuesday... For one single day I will consume water, black coffee, and cinnamon tea (sweetened with half a Splenda). I can and will do this because I can do anything in a day!	I DID IT!!!!!!!! I feel so strong, and I ate a healthy breakfast and got full very quickly :) I feel energetic and healthier— woohoo—great feeling! I'm going to do this every FIT Tuesday!	Normal Eating	Normal Eating	Normal Eating

FIGURE 23-3: Jenna's notes to herself during Week 1 to keep her motivated.

© John Wiley & Sons, Inc.

Create your own SMART goal weekly worksheet. Write down the five components (specific, measurable, attainable, realistic, and time-bound) like in Table 23-1 and record your own goals.

Your SMART goals don't have to be extraordinary feats. What they do have to be is doable *for you*. Choose a goal that is the best fit for you and you'll be much more likely to succeed if you set priorities that are compelling to you and feel attainable at present. Also, make sure you reward yourself every time you accomplish a SMART goal — a reward you can enjoy for a job well done — something as simple as taking 15 minutes to read a magazine, listening to your favorite music, or taking a soothing, luxurious bath.

Penciling in the Bigger Picture — Keeping Track of Why

You last tool in your toolbox is your long-term three-month health and wellness goal sheet. This exercise enables you to look at the bigger picture — the *why* you are practicing intermittent fasting. Always remembering why can help you stay motivated and not lose track of the real reasons you have chosen to make such a dramatic change in your lifestyle.

Begin by thinking about your whys. What is the real reason you're going on this journey? These are the big goals. Be honest with yourself about *why* making these dramatic lifestyle changes matter to you. Maybe it's for health reasons: You want to do this because you want to sleep better, improve your moods, or lower your blood pressure. Maybe it's for aesthetic reasons: You want to look better. Or maybe it's for personal reasons: You want to live longer and have more energy.

Begin by filling in the blanks. After three months, ask what you want the number on the scale to read. Consider health-related parameters, such as your blood pressure, your waist measurement, or anything else health-related such as "I will get my fasting blood sugar to under 100." Then add in a fitness goal, which can be a number or anything related to your fitness level, even something like: "I'll be able to walk one city block without stopping to rest."

Brian is a 28-year-old athletic man with no major health issues. He goes to the gym frequently and wants to change his diet and practice intermittent fasting to lose some body fat and add some muscle. He has a family history of heart disease, so he's concerned about his high cholesterol. Table 23-2 shows an example of Brian's three-month why sheet.

TABLE 23-2

Brian's Three-Month Goal Sheet

Parameter	Three-Month Goal
Weight	I will lose 5 pounds of body fat and gain 2 pounds of lean muscle.
Health	I will get my total cholesterol down to under 200 mg/dl.
Fitness	I will increase my deadlift weight from 310 pounds to 335 pounds.

Create your own three-month goal worksheet by specifying the three whys. Fill it out and refer back to it during your intermittent fast to keep you centered on your reasons wanting to get on and stay on this remarkable wellness program.

Chapter **24**

Getting Support during Your Intermittent Fast

oday's society can be harsh. You need to devote a substantial amount of conscious effort to maintaining a healthy body weight and staying physically fit. One of the best ways to stay on track and to have your new lifestyle behaviors sustain the test of time is to tap into those resources around you that can help you stay healthy and fit for life.

This chapter addresses the importance of getting help with your intermittent fasting efforts and offers numerous types of support you can access to help you on your intermittent fasting journey.

Getting Help from a Professional

There's nothing wrong with asking for professional help to reach your goals. You can access professionals and/or tracking devices that can aid your intermittent fasting experience. Your nutritionist can give you weekly tips and motivation to stay on track, helping you to overcome any obstacles and to set realistic goals. Here are some ideas of places to look:

>> **Personal nutrition consultant:** You can hire a registered dietitian/nutritionist for individualized nutrition advice.

To find a reputable nutritionist, look one up on the Academy of Nutrition and Dietetics website (www.eatright.org/). You can even find nutritionists that specialize in different areas. For instance, if you're a vegetarian, consult a member of the academy's vegetarian nutrition resource group at www.vndpg.org/home. If you're an athlete, consult with a certified specialist in sports dietetics at www.scandpg.org/home. If you want to focus on your weight, consult with a member of the weight management dietetics practice group at www.wmdpg.org/home. Fees can vary, but expect to pay about $150 for an initial visit and $75 for each follow-up visit.

>> **Personal trainer:** A personal trainer can help you with your exercise part of the intermittent fasting lifestyle equation. Just make sure that the trainer is certified by a reputable personal training certification organization.

Here are the five top organizations:

- American Council on Exercise (ACE) www.acefitness.org
- National Academy of Sports Medicine (NASM) www.nasm.org
- International Sports Sciences Association (ISSA) www.issaonline.com
- American College of Sports Medicine (ACSM) www.acsm.org
- National Strength and Conditioning Association (NSCA) www.nsca.com

>> **Nutrition and fitness apps:** Many health and fitness apps can help keep you on track and accountable (and some are free of charge!). In fact, studies show that people who use health and fitness apps are much more active compared to nonusers and have a lower body mass index (BMI; Chapter 2 discusses BMI). Here are my top five favorite apps:

- **MyFitnessPal:** This app is always a top-rated, easy-to-use app with a huge database and best of all, it's *free!*
- **Mindspace:** This app can help you reduce stress and get in your daily mindfulness/meditation exercise.
- **Aaptiv:** This workout app comes with your own trainer and an amazing playlist and gives you the ability to choose a workout based on the trainer, type of workout, duration, and music genre.
- **Viber:** This messaging app connects you with supportive online communities and groups. Online health and fitness communities are a great way to

help hold yourself accountable and seek motivation from like-minded individuals.

- **Seven:** This workout app for all level athletes allows you to customize the time and intensity of your exercise bout. The app authors suggest that seven minutes works for a quick strength-training workout. Sounds good to me!

Enlisting Friends and Family

Finding support for making difficult lifestyle changes can mean the difference between success and failure. Build your team with the people closest to you to give you support and make your behavior changes lasting at home, at work, and at social events. Studies have shown that having friends or family members who are supportive of your healthy eating and exercise goals is important for long-term success.

Keep in mind that support can come in many different types:

>> **Emotional support:** Someone to confide in when you're feeling discouraged

>> **Inspiring support:** Someone who encourages you to stick to it especially on days when your motivation may be waning

>> **Practical support:** Someone to help with the chores while you exercise or take some much-needed alone time

>> **Financial support:** Someone to help with the expense of hiring professional help

WARNING

Unfortunately, it's not uncommon to have some of your support network be unsupportive and critical. Some people push food on others, perhaps because they feel threatened by a person's perseverance. You may love these people, but they aren't your support team.

In fact, kids and spouses can be notorious deal-breakers.

>> To get your children on board, talk about the advantages of your intermittent fasting in sports nutrition language: better brainpower and more energy to work and play.

>> When talking to your spouse, mention things like more stamina, disease prevention, and graceful aging.

When organizing your support team, make sure to identify those people most helpful to you and weed out those least helpful. Establish your team around you because following an intermittent fasting lifestyle can be challenging, so find a support team that works to cheer you on and encourages you, no matter what!

TIP

Recognize the importance of giving and taking for your own success. Express your appreciation to your support team and be ready to return the favor and help others to get on the wellness journey. Helping others always gives you a return in kind. Gratitude is a thankful appreciation for what you receive, whether tangible or intangible. Gratitude will help you feel more positive emotions, relish good experiences, improve your health, deal with adversity, and build stronger relationships. Expressing daily gratitude is an important part of all wellness programs.

Dealing with Setbacks

You need to be aware that slips will occur over the long run, so go with the flow, and release any negative feelings of frustration, hopelessness, or failure, should they arise. Remember that nobody is perfect and that restructuring your thoughts from negative ones to positive ones is a healthy response. When you encounter a setback, don't dwell on it. Put it behind you, use it as a lesson, and get right back into your healthy intermittent fasting program. You can and will reach your highest goals if you stick with the plan.

Nearly everyone has had healthy eating and fitness setbacks or bumps in the road from time to time. Having a lapse and slipping into old patterns of behavior, particularly during stressful times, is just being a human.

Some people acknowledge these slips and bounce right back, using them as a signal to increase control. Others allow negative thoughts (guilt or frustration) to take over, leading to loss of control. A collection of lapses, such that you fall back into old habits for an extended period of time, is called a *relapse*. Everyone has lapses; it's the relapse that you should try and avoid. You can take action to prevent a relapse by staying aware, keeping at your plan with your goals in mind, and staying positive.

REMEMBER

The important lesson: You can't control everything in your life; what you can control is how you respond to those lapses. Don't beat yourself up. Pick yourself up, shake off the dust, and get right back on it. Here are some preventative setback strategies for you to keep up your sleeve:

TIP

>> **Keep journaling.** Regardless of whether you stay on track or go off course, journaling helps with awareness.

Make sure to hold onto and use your journals and completed goal sheets as tools to help you in the future. By memorializing your past successes and failures, you can see for yourself what is working and what isn't. Refer to Chapter 23 for more information about journaling.

>> **Plan in advance.** If you know a difficult situation is coming up, plan ahead. If your power business lunch is during your fasting time, perhaps you may want to switch to another intermittent fast for that week. You can also prepare for special events like a birthday party or family gathering by planning ahead. Going out and eating healthy food options is already hard enough, but going out to eat, and not having the option to eat at all? Intermittent fasting doesn't leave room for a social life, unless you schedule your dates around your nonfasting days.

>> **Look at the restaurant's menu online.** Study the restaurant's menu online beforehand and ensure that that restaurant serves healthy fare. If you're following the 5:2 intermittent fast, you can do the calorie calculations and come up with what you'll eat and drink to stay within your calorie range.

>> **Analyze your behavior chain.** Write down what led you to go off your intermittent fast. Jot down the actions you took before, during, and after your lapse so that you can identify the behavior chain. See where you could have broken the chain so you can be aware of future lapses.

>> **Weigh yourself.** As difficult as it may be, you can use the scale to your advantage. If you gained weight, put a positive spin on it, using your feelings to instigate control. Take back control and empower yourself.

>> **Keep a graph.** If you write down what was happening in your life during times of weight loss or weight gain, you'll get a much clearer view of how your behaviors affect your body. Chapter 23 explains how you can incorporate graphing into your plan to measure your progress.

>> **Read some old journals.** To get back on track, pull out some old journals or goal sheets and see where you reached your weekly goal. Study them and repeat those behaviors that worked for you in the past.

>> **Think positive.** Look at how far you have come and all the positive changes that you have made. Remember, nobody is perfect. You can do it.

7

The Part of Tens

Break apart the common myths about intermittent fasting.

Unearth the top superfoods to add into your eating windows.

Chapter 25

Ten Myths about Intermittent Fasting Debunked

Like many other diet trends, intermittent fasting has taken on an identity of its own. The media has exploded with information about the unlimited benefits of intermittent fasting. But are the claims true? This chapter examines ten of the most common myths about fasting and debunks each one.

Intermittent Fasting Puts Your Body Into Starvation Mode

Intermittent fasting isn't starving but an occasional planned break in food intake for relatively short time periods, done voluntarily for health and wellness purposes. One common myth of intermittent fasting is that it puts your body into starvation mode, thus shutting down your metabolism. People who are starving do so involuntarily, when food is scarce such as during times of famine and war. Prolonged calorie restriction can cause the body to adapt to the lack of intake and go into a *starvation mode,* which means the body severely reduces metabolic rate as a survival technique. Intermittent fasting is a far cry from starvation.

REMEMBER

Intermittent fasting prevents the starvation mode adaptation by regularly alternating between consumption and restriction. In fact, limiting the fasting period and alternating between fasting and feasting *increases* metabolic rate. Studies reveal that fasting for up to 48 hours can boost metabolism by 4 to 14 percent. However, if you fast much longer, the effects can reverse, decreasing your metabolism.

Skipping Breakfast Makes You Fat

According to Mom, breakfast is the most important meal of the day. Although that may be true for some people, research has shown that breakfast isn't essential for your health. Controlled studies don't show any difference in weight loss between those individuals who eat breakfast and those who skip it.

REMEMBER

You aren't slowing down your metabolism by skipping breakfast. On the contrary, intermittent fasting has been shown to significantly boost your metabolic rate and promote loss of body fat.

Intermittent Fasting Slows Metabolism and Frequent Meals Boost It

Eating smaller, more frequent meals doesn't boost your metabolism a significant amount or help you lose weight. In fact, what matters most is the total number of calories you consume — not how many meals you eat.

TECHNICAL STUFF

Regarding small, frequent meals, without question, your body does indeed expend some calories digesting meals — the scientific term is the *thermic effect of food (TEF).* On average, the TEF uses around 10 percent of your total calorie intake, which is a negligible boost in metabolism.

New research on intermittent fasting has proven that flipping your metabolic switch, for short time periods, *revs up your metabolism* by decreasing insulin levels and boosting blood levels of human growth hormone and norepinephrine. These changes can help you burn fat more easily and help you lose weight. One study showed that fasting every other day for 22 days didn't lead to a reduction in metabolic rate but did result in a 4 percent loss of fat mass.

Eating Three Meals a Day Is Better for Your Health

Some people believe that the standard pattern of eating three meals a day plus snacks is better for health and weight control, but doing so is just not true. Instead, fasting from time to time has major health benefits. The three-meal-a-day-plus-snacks lifestyle doesn't induce the physiological changes in the body proven to promote the magical *autophagy* process (the cellular repair process). Short-term fasting induces autophagy so your cells recycle old and dysfunctional proteins. Autophagy may help protect against aging, cancer, and neurodegenerative conditions like Parkinson's and Alzheimer's disease. In fact, some studies even suggest that snacking or eating very often harms your health and *raises* your risk of disease. Hence, intermittent fasting is far from unhealthy — and offers numerous benefits not seen with the traditional eating pattern.

You Need to Eat Protein Every Three Hours to Gain Muscle

Studies show that eating your protein in more frequent doses doesn't affect muscle mass. The idea that you need to eat protein every couple of hours and also eat 20 to 30 grams of protein with each meal and snack for muscle gain is untrue. People can gain muscle and lose body fat when intermittent fasting. The key is to eat before and after your strength-training workouts and get in enough total calories (and protein) for muscle gain.

REMEMBER

A program of weight training geared to muscle gain during intermittent fasting and consuming enough calories to support muscle growth is the key to gaining muscle. Your body can easily make use of more than 30 grams of protein per meal. You *don't* need to consume protein every two to three hours.

Intermittent Fasting Makes You Lose Muscle

Some people believe that when you fast, your body starts cannibalizing its own muscle for energy. Strict low-calorie diets do promote loss of body fat and lean body mass, which is why intermittent fasting programs promote a gradual loss of a maximum of 2 pounds per week — combined with a resistance exercise program — so you lose the fat and retain the muscle. Strategic intermittent fasting preserves and protects muscle mass rather than breaking it down.

REMEMBER

In fact, some studies show that intermittent fasting is better for maintaining muscle mass compared to conventional dieting. One study showed a modest increase in muscle mass for people who followed the Warrior intermittent fasting plan and consumed all their calories during one huge meal in the evening (see Chapter 10 for more about the Warrior plan).

Notably, intermittent fasting is popular among many bodybuilders who frequently practice it to maintain muscle mass along with an extremely low percentage of body fat. The proven release of growth hormone during the fasted state is clearly an attractive side effect of intermittent fasting for this group of athletes. Many bodybuilders have started intermittent fasting because they know that adopting periods of intermittent fasting helps them achieve their primary goals: burn excess fat and retain lean muscle.

Intermittent Fasting Triggers Excessive Hunger and Makes You Overeat

Study after study proves intermittent fasting to be a highly effective weight loss method. And no evidence suggests intermittent fasting promotes weight gain. That's not to say that if you gorge and overeat during your feasting periods that you won't gain weight — you absolutely will. That being said, intermittent fasting is a powerful tool for weight loss because of the metabolic changes that occur in the body such as a reduction in insulin levels while at the same time a boost in metabolism, norepinephrine levels, and human growth hormone levels, so you lose fat — not gain it. The bottom line, though, is that you lose weight because you successfully create a *calorie deficit*, where you eat less calories and expend more, over time. (If you upend this equation, you will gain weight.)

However if you follow the plan like it's designed, over time, usually two to four weeks, your body adapts to the hunger feelings and you actually become less hungry and are satisfied with less food. Life hurts. Life is suffering, the Buddha said. Lawrence of Arabia said the trick is . . . not minding that it hurts.

TIP

Put a positive spin on the hunger pangs. Imagine the fat evaporating away. When you lose weight, most of your fat is converted to the gases carbon dioxide and water vapor, and so you get rid of fat by breathing it out of your body.

Intermittent Fasting Is Harmful to the Brain

The brain does thrive on blood sugar (also known as glucose), its preferred fuel. However, eating carbs every few hours is totally unnecessary for brain health for a couple of reasons:

>> Your body can easily create new glucose from non-carbohydrate sources via a process called *gluconeogenesis*.

>> During your fasted state, the brain uses ketones as an alternate energy source that precludes the need to provide the brain with a constant dietary glucose intake.

By forcing your body to burn its fat reserves and run on ketones intermittently, you'll not only keep your brain going during those periods of fasting but you'll also improve cognition, grow the connections between neurons, and stave off neurodegeneration. Chapter 6 provides more details about this process.

Intermittent Fasting Causes Dangerous Drops in Blood Sugar

Intermittent fasting actually stabilizes blood sugar levels and helps to prevent and potentially reverse type 2 diabetes. Your body is a glucose-storing and glucose-making machine. Glucose levels typically stabilize, and over time the body goes through tremendous improvements and even reversal of insulin-resistant conditions like diabetes with strategic intermittent fasts.

WARNING

Hypoglycemia (abnormally low blood glucose) is only a precaution in people previously diagnosed with this disorder and in diabetics if they're taking insulin or oral pills that lower glucose. In these situations, you must get permission to follow an intermittent fast from your healthcare professional. She'll need to closely supervise you and monitor your glucose levels if you're incorporating intermittent fasting. Chapter 7 discusses blood sugar and diabetics in more detail.

Intermittent Fasting Is Too Hard

Intermittent fasting can be challenging. Yet most people agree that it's much easier than traditional diets. It doesn't involve any tedious caloric tracking (you're either eating or not), making it a much more manageable weight loss method for many people.

Furthermore, your sacrifice yields countless rewards not seen in old-style dieting: health benefits and weight and fat loss. In addition, you have freedom from food restrictions during your eating windows. Eating less frequently means exerting far less time and energy thinking about food, shopping for food, and cooking food. As a result, you spend more time on the things you enjoy in life. Check out Chapter 6 for the miraculous health benefits that come from intermittent fasting to help you get the motivation and continue on with your intermittent fasting journey of choice with the knowledge that you *can* do it!

Chapter **26**

Ten Healthiest Superfoods to Include When Intermittent Fasting

This chapter discusses ten beautiful, crazy-healthy superfoods that you can add to your intermittent fasting lifestyle!

With intermittent fasting you are when you eat *and* what you eat.

REMEMBER You may notice that all the foods on this superfood list are plants. Hot off the presses is a new mega-study published in the *British Medical Journal* showing that eating mostly plant protein reduces your risk of death. Diets high in plant protein, such as legumes (peas, beans, and lentils), whole grains, and nuts reduce risks of developing diabetes, heart disease, and stroke, whereas regular consumption of red meat and a high intake of animal proteins has been linked to several health problems and a shorter life. Tap into the power of plants for a longer, healthier, leaner life!

All of these foods contain Mother Nature's medicine chest called phytochemicals. *Phytochemicals* describes the thousands of nutrients found in edible plants that play a major role in preventing degenerative disease such as heart disease and cancer. Phytochemicals (*phyto* is Greek for *plant*) are found in fruits, vegetables, whole grains, and other plant foods. Chapter 17 discusses phytochemicals in more detail.

Black Coffee

I can't say enough about the health and weight loss benefits of drinking black coffee. Coffee beans are seeds, and like all seeds, they're loaded with protective plant compounds. In fact, coffee is the single greatest source of antioxidants in the Western diet. I call it "plant juice." Note that decaf coffee contains similar amounts of antioxidants as regular coffee. Purchase organic coffee when possible, better for you and the environment. As a bonus, organic coffee beans are richer in healthful antioxidants and chlorogenic acid, which are helpful in preventing type 2 diabetes and lowering blood pressure. Many people can even taste the difference. Your health, and the health of the planet, both get a boost.

TIP

Drive through your favorite barista bar and order a large dark roast with a shot of espresso (decaf if the caffeine doesn't agree with you). Make it iced for an antioxidant-packed cold brew.

Spinach

Spinach is a nutritional powerhouse. This nutrient-dense green superfood is readily available — fresh, frozen, or even canned. One of the healthiest foods on the planet, spinach is super low in calories yet packed with nutrients such as vitamin C, vitamin A, vitamin K, potassium, and essential folate. It's also loaded with potassium and magnesium — minerals that lower blood pressure.

WARNING

The Environmental Working Groups *Shopper's Guide to Pesticides in Produce* ranks spinach second on its list of fruits and vegetables with the most pesticides. Refer to Chapter 18 for more about this list. Buy organic to avoid the pesticides.

TIP

I prefer to buy plain frozen spinach because one cup of frozen spinach has more than four times the amount of nutrients, such as fiber, folate, iron, and calcium than a cup of fresh spinach.

Quinoa

Loaded with vitamins, minerals, antioxidants, and fiber, quinoa (KEEN-wah) is incredibly nutritious. It's also unique among grains because it's a complete protein, meaning it contains the right amount of all essential amino acids your body needs to build new proteins. In fact, quinoa has twice the protein of regular cereal grains.

REMEMBER

Quinoa is a whole grain. For optimal health, you need to eat more whole grains and much less refined grains. Chapter 17 examines what a whole grain is and how you can easily spot one.

TIP

Serve quinoa as a substitute for rice, especially refined white rice (it cooks much quicker and comes out light and fluffy) or even in salads. Most grocery stores now carry it in the rice and beans aisle.

Extra-Virgin Olive Oil (EVOO)

Extra-virgin olive oil (EVOO) is loaded with antioxidants and healthy fats and has been shown to offer numerous health benefits. EVOO is the only vegetable oil that contains a large amount of disease-fighting polyphenols and anti-inflammatory substances. Chronic inflammation is believed to be among the leading drivers of many diseases, including heart disease, cancer, metabolic syndrome, diabetes, and arthritis. Refer to Chapter 17 for loads more information on EVOO.

TIP

Keep a small dark bottle of authentic EVOO with a pour spout near your cooktop. Drizzle, don't douse your food because olive oil, like all fat, is calorie dense. Use just a touch of EVOO whenever you sauté foods in your skillet.

Black Beans

Beans were known as peasant food, poor man's meat but are now known as a healthy person's staple. Unfortunately, Americans have failed to embrace beans — a tasty, versatile, hearty, and ridiculously inexpensive superfood. Beans contain the most protein of any vegetable; plus, they're loaded with essential B vitamins (especially the heart-healthy folate), minerals, and fiber to help you feel full longer. Beans are also a rich source of complex carbohydrates that provide long-lasting energy, good slow carbs.

The dark varieties of beans such as black beans, top the U.S. Department of Agriculture's list of foods highest in disease-fighting antioxidants. These little black beauties are packed with nutrients such as calcium, plant protein, and fiber, and they also taste great! Black beans can fill you up without draining your wallet, and now they're trendier than ever. A lean plant protein, black beans should be on everyone's plate a few times a week. Chapter 8 delves more into the benefits of eating beans.

TIP

Buy low-sodium, canned beans, rinse several times, and then dry the beans and add to salads or make quick tacos or a burrito.

Beets

Good for the brain and potent at lowering blood pressure, the humble beet is often overlooked as one of the healthiest foods on earth. Beets boast an impressive nutritional profile —low in calories, yet dense with valuable nutrients such as fiber, folate, manganese, potassium, calcium, iron, and vitamin C. Beets also provide a good dose of nitrates. (Your body changes nitrates into *nitric oxide,* a chemical that helps lower blood pressure and improve athletic performance.)

Choose the red/purple variety to protect your cells from free radical damage by consuming a daily dose of a polyphenol flavonoid called anthocyanins — the blue pigmented polyphenol found in red/purple beets. Beets are naturally low in sodium and are virtually fat and cholesterol free. Beets generally show low pesticide residues, and therefore are generally okay to buy non-organic.

TIP

Buy the packaged pre-cooked and peeled version, slice, and throw into your salad. Or peel, douse with EVOO, and roast them. This will retain the good-for-you phytonutrients that leach out of the food and into the water if boiled extensively.

Nuts and Seeds

Walnuts, almonds, and pistachios (raw and unsalted) as well as chia seeds and ground flaxseeds are all true superfoods. Essential fatty acids are required in the diet for optimal health. Both nuts and seeds are bursting with these essential good fats, called *omega-3 alpha-linolenic acid (ALA).* Walnuts and flaxseeds are two ancient plant foods that have sustained humans since the birth of civilization — and both are top sources of ALA. In addition, nuts and seeds are antioxidant powerhouses. Chapter 17 discusses nuts and seeds in more detail.

TIP

Keep a supply of nuts in your bag for an easy, healthy snacks. Or, packets of single serving on-the-go chia and ground flaxseeds are available for purchase in most health food stores or online (toss them in smoothies or in cereal).

Broccoli

Broccoli is a nutritional powerhouse full of vitamins (especially vitamin C), minerals, fiber, and antioxidants. Broccoli belongs to the plant species known as *Brassica oleracea*. Broccoli, Brussels sprouts, kale, and cauliflower — all edible plants — collectively are referred to as cruciferous vegetables. Researchers have shown that this group of vegetables, also known as the anti-cancer vegetables, can effectively treat dysfunction of the arteries and heart vessel damage in diabetics.

Cruciferous vegetables are natural cancer-prevention foods, that should be consumed most days of the week. Low in calories and rich in fiber, broccoli is the perfect super-healthy addition to your feasting periods. Don't worry about paying more for organic. Broccoli generally doesn't end up with pesticide residue. Vegetables, such as broccoli, promote healthy gut flora — rich in prebiotics or food for healthy gut bacteria. Prebiotics also can boost the diversity of your good gut bugs.

TIP

Steam your broccoli for the most vitamin preservation. Squirt butter spray (25 sprays is a mere 20 calories) for flavor and enjoy as a side dish.

Blackberries

Berries, in general, are the ultimate anti-aging superfood. In particular, blackberries contain a wide array of important nutrients including potassium, magnesium and calcium, as well as vitamins A, C, E, calcium, iron, and most of the B vitamins. They're also a rich source of anthocyanins that give blackberries their deep purple color.

Just one cup of raw blackberries has 60 calories, 30 milligrams of vitamin C, and a megadose of 8 grams of dietary fiber (one serving of blackberries delivers 31 percent of your daily dietary fiber needs). Fresh or frozen, blackberries are a true superfood that deserves a spot on your weekly menu. I suggest purchasing organic, if available.

TIP

Sprinkle them on yogurt or eat plain as a sweet and delicious snack. Blackberries also work well in smoothies.

Lentils

The mighty legume is high in fiber and protein and adds great taste and texture to any meal. Vegans and vegetarians are often a fan of using lentils as a meat substitute in traditional recipes; only unlike animal protein, lentils are fat and cholesterol free. Lentils are made up of more than 25 percent protein. They're also a great source of iron, a mineral that is sometimes lacking in vegetarian diets. Lentils are inexpensive, cook quickly and easily, and are low in calories, rich in iron and folate, and an excellent source of additional nutrients.

Lentils require no soaking, and they cook in a reasonable amount of time, anywhere from 10 to 25 minutes depending on the variety. You can also buy precooked lentils, which taste great and speed prep.

TIP

Add cooked lentils to your tomato sauce for extra protein, fiber, and taste. Lentils pack enough meaty flavor to make a Bolognese sauce taste like the real thing. Chopped bell peppers add another layer of texture, and a thick tomato paste makes it deliciously saucy.

Index

Numbers

guided imagery, 143

gut microbiome

  eat-stop-eat plan and, 129–130

  intermittent fasting and, 76–77

  ketogenic diet and, 101

  prebiotics and, 295

H

HA (carcinogenic heterocyclic amines), 209–210

"hangry," 110, 146. *See also* emotions; mood

HDL cholesterol, 50, 83, 129, 135, 141

headaches, 149–150

healthy weight

  calculating

    BMI, 27–29

    body fat measurements, 31–32

    discussion, 25

    via scale, 25–26

    waist measurements, 29–30

    weight formulas, 26–27

  mood and, 21

heart disease

  ADF and, 121

  black coffee and, 96

  excess fat and, 53

  exercise and, 135

  fat storage patterns and, 29–30

  obesity and, 47

  overabundance and, 80

  visceral fat and, 55

hemp seeds, 172

herbal teas, 95, 98

high blood pressure

  decreasing, 75

  obesity and, 22, 47, 53

  sleep and, 68

  strength training and, 141

Hofmekler, Ori, 112

human growth hormone (HGH), 62, 71, 74, 129, 138

hunger

  cravings versus, 161–162

  discussion, 15, 88

fears related to, 146

  mood and, 109–110

  myths regarding, 288

hunter-gatherers, 14, 16, 71

hydration, 9, 84, 148, 150

hyperglycemia, 75

hypoglycemia, 86–87, 150, 289

I

icons, 3

inflammation

  ADF and, 120

  exercise and, 134

  ketones and, 65

  obesity and, 50

  plant-based foods and, 178

  reducing, 76

  sleep and, 68

  visceral fat and, 55, 73

insomnia, 88

insulin, 51, 64, 71

insulin resistance

  ADF and, 119

  decreasing, 61, 75

  exercise and, 134–135

  obesity and, 48, 53

  type 2 diabetes and, 86

  in women, 51

insulin sensitivity

  ADF and, 120–121

  increased, 61, 86, 109, 137

  sleep and, 67

  strength training and, 141

intermittent fasting. *See also* calories; cardiovascular exercise; exercise; fasting; mind-body exercises; *specific forms of intermittent fasting*

  adjusting to, 43–44, 83–84

  benefits of

    decreased insulin resistance, 75

    decreased risk of diabetes, 75

    fat loss, 75

    increased autophagy, 77, 80

    increased cognition, 79

    mental health, 77

overview, 11–13, 74

    reduced high blood pressure, 75

    reduced inflammation, 76

    reduced oxidative stress, 75, 78–79

    weight loss, 75

  diabetics and

    comparing types, 85

    overview, 84–86

    risks, 86–87

  difficulties during

    fatigue, 148–149

    food cravings, 146–147

    headaches, 149–150

    hunger fears, 146

    overview, 145

    scheduling conflicts, 150–151

  ease of following, 1, 12

  foods to include in

    beets, 294

    black beans, 293–294

    black coffee, 292

    blackberries, 295–296

    broccoli, 242, 295

    EVOO, 293

    lentils, 296

    nuts and seeds, 294–295

    overview, 291–292

    quinoa, 293

    spinach, 292

  goals in, 2, 93–94

  key principles, 9–10

  metabolic states in, 63–66

  myths regarding

    blood sugar drop, 289

    cognitive function, 289

    fasting too difficult, 290

    hunger, 288

    meal frequency, 287

    muscle mass loss, 288

    overview, 285

    skipping breakfast, 286

  not mixing keto diet with, 100–103

  physiological effects of, 59–62, 67

  preparation for, 16–17

  questions regarding, 15–16

T

TDEE (total daily energy expenditure), 38–39

testosterone, 141

thermic effect of food (TEF), 35–36, 38, 286

thyroid hormone, 74, 88

time-restricted plan. *See* intermittent fasting

TMA (trimethylamine), 130

TMAO (trimethylamine N-oxide), 129–130

total daily energy expenditure (TDEE), 38–39

traditional fasting, 8–9, 71

trans fats, 189

triglycerides
- ADF and, 120
- from being overweight, 50
- discussion, 74, 76, 83
- eat-stop-eat plan and, 129
- exercise and, 135
- nuts and, 179

triiodothyronine, 119

trimethylamine (TMA), 130

trimethylamine N-oxide (TMAO), 129–130

type 1 diabetes, 10, 85–86

type 2 diabetes
- black coffee and, 97
- compared with type 1 diabetes, 85
- discussion, 10, 45, 75
- excess fat and, 54
- exercise and, 134
- overabundance and, 80
- sleep and, 68
- visceral fat and, 55

U

underwater weighing, 31

unhealthy foods, 9, 37–38, 52. *See also* empty calorie foods

V

Varady, Krista, 120

vegans, 172, 229. *See also* recipes

vegetables
- discussion, 169, 183, 200
- from farmers' markets, 185–186
- organic, 193–194

vegetarians, 172, 229. *See also* recipes

visceral fat
- appetite and, 55
- cardiovascular exercise and, 134
- discussion, 1–2, 29, 53–54
- mood and, 55
- risks related to, 55, 73
- type 2 diabetes and, 86

W

waist measurements, 29–30, 271–273

Warrior Diet, The (Hofmekler), 112

warrior eating plan
- balancing calorie intake in, 112
- discussion, 13, 106, 111
- exercising during, 114
- OMAD versus, 113
- pros and cons of, 113
- sample 1-week, 115

water, 95, 150

weight. *See* healthy weight

weight formulas, 26–27

weight gain, 34–35, 37

weight loss. *See also* calories; healthy weight
- ADF and, 120
- benefits of, 20–22, 46
- calorie deficit and
  - 80:20 rule, 42–43
  - calculating daily needs, 40–42
  - food choices, 37–38
  - overview, 36–37, 106, 288

discussion, 1–2, 13, 19

exercise and, 37, 134

ideal rate of, 72

muscle mass maintenance during, 71–73

promoted by intermittent fasting, 70–71

role of hormones in, 62

tips for permanent, 66

via sustainable caloric deficit, 70–71

weight scale, 25–26

whole foods diet, 99–100, 103. *See also* Mediterranean Diet

whole grains
- bran in, 175–176
- discussion, 102–103, 169, 184, 200
- endosperm in, 175–176
- finding, 176–178
- germ in, 175–176
- in Mediterranean Diet, 174–176

Wilks, James, 114

women
- 500-calorie recipes for
  - Cajun Grilled Chicken, 255
  - Cheesy Bean Burrito, 258
  - Farro Salad, 257
  - Honey-Crusted Salmon with Spinach, 256
  - overview, 253
  - Whole Grain Linguini with Cannellini Beans, 259
- essential fats in, 31
- fast diet plan and, 123
- fat storage patterns in, 53–54
- waist measurements in, 30
- weight formulas for, 26–27

Y

yoga, 143–144

About the Author

Janet Bond Brill, PhD, RDN, FAND, was born and raised in New York City, the daughter of a prominent stage and screen actor and a psychoanalyst. At the age of 16, she graduated Walden School in Manhattan and enrolled at the University of Miami. After earning her bachelor's degree in biology she took a break from academia and traveled the world, working as a flight attendant for Pan American World Airways. Returning to South Florida, she earned both her doctoral degree and master's degree in exercise physiology from the University of Miami, in addition to a second master's degree in nutrition science from Florida International University, graduating both universities with academic honors. She has taught both graduate and undergraduate courses in nutrition, health, and fitness as an adjunct professor at the University of Miami, Florida International University, and Cedar Crest College.

Dr. Janet has become a nationally recognized nutrition, health, and fitness expert and has authored three books: *Blood Pressure DOWN, Prevent a Second Heart Attack*, and *Cholesterol DOWN* (all by Random House). She is a prolific writer with contributions to numerous scientific journals and lay publications worldwide. Currently, Dr. Janet writes a column for Bottom Line Health, Inc.

She is a trusted source of information for the national media and is a frequent guest expert on local and national television. Nationally, she has appeared on the Dr. Oz show numerous times, CBS "On the Couch," and as a nutrition expert for "The Balancing Act" (Lifetime). On a personal note, she has completed four marathons and countless road races, many for charitable organizations. A dedicated mother of three fantastic children and a devoted wife of 36 years, Dr. Janet and her family reside in Allentown, Pennsylvania.

Dr. Janet believes whole-heartedly in the role both good nutrition and exercise play in the prevention of chronic disease and achieving optimal health. She teaches the importance of a healthy lifestyle and has helped thousands of people across the nation improve their health and wellbeing.

Dedication

I dedicate this book to my parents-in-law, Edna Stefania Brill and Harry Brill. Sadly, Edna and Harry passed away just this past year. Both Edna and Harry were Holocaust survivors, having endured unspeakable and unimaginable horrors early in life. Yet their ability to transcend the trauma and go on to live rich and fulfilling lives are testaments to their extraordinary resilience, strength, and will to live that will forever be etched in my mind and those lucky enough to have had them in their lives. They were kind, generous people without whom I couldn't have received the education that has catapulted my career. Thank you, dear Edna and Harry, for giving me your son and for being the most loving grandparents in the world to my children, for which I'm so very grateful. A bright light had been extinguished from this earth but will live on through eternity in my heart. Rest in peace, my dear mother and father.

Author Acknowledgments

To Margot Hutchinson of Waterside Productions, who was my source for connecting me to Wiley, enabling me to write this book. Thank you, Margot. To my colleagues at Wiley: Acquisition Editor Tracy Boggier who has been very helpful in keeping this project on course. Much appreciation also goes to my Project Editor and Copy Editor Chad Sievers, thank you for your excellent insight and invaluable help in creating this book.

Many thanks to Bari Bossis for her help with the recipes.

To my family: Sam, Rachel, Mia, Jeremy, and Jason who supported my writing this book during the excruciating stress of the pandemic. Thank you and remember that you are and will always be, my everything.

And to my 97-year-old mother, Dr. Alma Halbert Bond, who is healthier and sharper than I am! Thank you for your inspiration and showing me that a woman can do it all — family, work, marriage, and good health and fitness for life by taking care of one's body with diet and exercise.

Publisher's Acknowledgments

Senior Acquisitions Editor: Tracy Boggier

Project Editor: Chad R. Sievers

Technical Editor: Kristina M. LaRue, RDN

Production Editor: Mohammed Zafar Ali

Cover Image: © Kreminska/Shutterstock